The Friendship Blueprint

The Friendship Blueprint provides those committed to empowering young people to thrive with an evidence informed pathway to profoundly impact student capability, social culture, and healthy relationships. Pro social skills are not acquired with automaticity, nor are they easy to apply while navigating social glitches with a developmentally immature and reactive primary school and adolescent brain; where emotions and impulses reign over logic and perspective. In a world where social connection is the foundation of happiness and achievement, mastering friendship skills is no longer optional, it's essential.

Packed with practical strategies, engaging stories, and step-by-step activities, *The Friendship Blueprint* equips children with the tools to build strong, supportive relationships at home, in school, and beyond. Each chapter offers actionable lessons, reflection prompts, and real-world scenarios that make complex social skills accessible and fun. Special features include posters, case studies, and extension activities that foster empathy, communication, and resilience, preparing learners for challenges inside and outside the classroom.

The Friendship Blueprint isn't just a book, it's a curriculum for life. Invest in children's emotional intelligence and set them on a path toward academic, personal, and career success by empowering them with the skills that matter most.

Madhavi Nawana Parker is the CEO of Positive Minds Australia, a widely published author, keynote speaker, podcast and radio guest, whose specialisation in social emotional wellbeing, student engagement, compassionate leadership, and connected parenting has been acknowledged through global nominations and awards over the past three decades. Madhavi lives in South Australia and is married with three children.

"In an era of rising loneliness, post-pandemic social delays, and increasing digital distraction, Madhavi Nawana Parker has created a rich curriculum with the essential, evidence-based social-emotional skills urgently needed to build real connection, resilience, and lifelong wellbeing in students."

Emma McKenzie, *School Counsellor, Prince Alfred College, SA*

"Friendships and genuine connections shape a young person's sense of identity, belonging and mattering. The explicit teaching of these skills is vital, and with Madhavi's deep expertise leading the way, *The Friendship Blueprint* offers a clear and practical path for educators and families to help every child grow into capable, connected and caring learners."

Emily Rogers, *Assistant Head of McGregor Campus, Seymour College, SA*

"In classrooms every day, we observe first hand the impact of friendships on learning and wellbeing. *The Friendship Blueprint*'s social and emotional intelligence tools equip educators with a curriculum to help all students thrive."

Sarah Shoobridge, *Head of Teaching and Development, Scotch College, SA*

"*The Friendship Blueprint*, offers practical, research-informed skills - empathy, emotional regulation, communication, and inclusion - that help young people navigate social challenges with confidence and care. Madhavi's work strengthens connection and supports schools to create environments where every child can truly thrive."

David Kolpak, *Principal Trinity College North School, SA*

"Nawana Parker understands that young people cannot learn unless they feel connected, safe, and resilient. Her practical, evidence-based strategies and real-world anecdotes provide an essential blueprint for educational leaders seeking to meet the diverse needs of their students."

Lee Del Col, *Christian Brothers College, SA*

The Friendship Blueprint

The Power of Social Connection for School, Family, and Career Success

Madhavi Nawana Parker

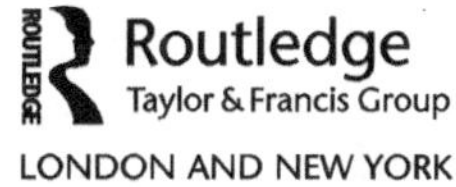

Routledge
Taylor & Francis Group

LONDON AND NEW YORK

Book cover layout and illustrations by Rachel Reiter

First published 2027
by Routledge
4 Park Square, Milton Park, Abingdon, Oxon OX14 4RN

and by Routledge
605 Third Avenue, New York, NY 10158

Routledge is an imprint of the Taylor & Francis Group, an informa business

British Library Cataloguing-in-Publication Data
A catalogue record for this book is available from the British Library

ISBN: 978-1-041-02059-2 (hbk)
ISBN: 978-1-041-02057-8 (pbk)
ISBN: 978-1-003-61757-0 (ebk)

DOI: 10.4324/9781003617570

Typeset in Optima LT Std
by KnowledgeWorks Global Ltd.

*The Friendship Blueprint is dedicated to my parents,
the late Srinath and Mallika Nawana, my first friends.
You showed me how to be a friend, by being a friend,
not just to me, but to everyone. Your lessons are with me,
in every beat of my heart. Thank you.*

Contents

Contents

8 Being yourself in friendships: Authenticity matters **201**

9 Choosing the right friends and navigating social roadblocks **226**

Foreword

Friendship is one of the most profound gifts we can offer and receive. Like the humans who form them, friendships are wonderfully complex, shaping the way we see the world around us and also ourselves. In schools, families, and communities, these connections become the foundation upon which children and young people build their understanding of belonging, identity, and purpose.

This book offers a timely and thoughtful exploration of how the core skills of social and emotional learning—self-awareness, empathy, regulation, communication, and inclusion—can be nurtured through the everyday experiences of friendship. It recognises that well-being and learning are inseparable. As educators and leaders, we witness this truth daily: when friendships flourish, so too do resilience, positive self-concept, and confidence. As a teacher and educational leader for 35 years and parent for 24 of those years, I have seen first-hand that for children and young people, especially, healthy friendships cultivated alongside self-awareness become pathways to greater life satisfaction and a deeper sense of meaning and connection.

Yet today's children and young people navigate friendship in a landscape vastly different from previous generations. Social media has fundamentally reshaped how connections are formed, maintained, and sometimes fractured, bringing both unprecedented opportunities for connection and genuine new challenges. The curated nature of online profiles, the pressure of constant availability, and the permanence of digital interactions have introduced new dimensions to the experience of friendship itself.

In Australia, the social media ban for children under 16, due to take effect in late 2025, represents a significant moment in how we collectively respond to these challenges. This legislation acknowledges both the potential harms of early social media exposure and the importance of protecting the developmental space where face-to-face friendship skills are nurtured. It underscores a question many of us are grappling with: how do we help children develop authentic, resilient friendships in an age where digital and physical worlds increasingly intertwine? We might ask our young people a simple question: would you rather have 500 followers who scroll past your posts, or two friends who notice when you are unusually quiet? The answer reveals what we all know deep down—that authentic friendship is not measured in cursory clicks, but in genuine care. This book arrives at a crucial time, offering guidance that honours both the timeless foundations of friendship and the realities young people navigate today.

What makes this book particularly valuable is the practical wisdom woven throughout each chapter. Written by a respected colleague, true friend, and treasured source of positivity to me and many others, Madhavi brings together insight, warmth, and accessibility in equal measure. Readers will explore how to handle big feelings, protect their friendship battery, and embrace their authentic selves. Central to this journey is a liberating truth: being a good friend is not about being perfect. It is about listening, caring, and learning from each other through both the smooth moments and the stumbles.

Whether you are a teacher seeking to foster more inclusive classrooms, a parent guiding your child through the complexities of social life, or a young person eager to understand the dynamics of your own friendships, this book will speak to you. It is both a guide and an invitation: to reflect deeply, to act with courage and compassion, and to embrace the adventure of friendship as a lifelong journey. In these pages, you will find not only knowledge, but also encouragement—a reminder that the work of building strong, healthy friendships is among the most important and rewarding endeavours we undertake as humans.

I commend this book to you. May it inspire connection, nurture empathy, and equip readers of all ages with the tools to create relationships that sustain and uplift us all.

Anne Dunstan
Chief Executive
Association of Independent Schools of South Australia

Preface

Phenomenal friendships, impactful connections with teachers, and a family to love with all my heart were my saving grace through primary and high school. Without them, the sudden loss of my Dad to Leukemia when he was just 45 and I was 10, combined with constant, daily struggles with attention, focus, learning, and grief could have destroyed me. Relationships are everything.

After nearly 30 years working in education and well-being, I've witnessed first-hand, the profound impact that friendship and connection have. My career has taken me into homes where generational trauma bled out through the walls and into classrooms, where children ached to the core with loneliness, hopelessness, and helplessness. I've sat with thousands of exemplary and inspirational educators and parents scratching their heads doing everything they can, to bring hope back into the lives of disconnected young people to prove to them, how much their lives matter. I've watched children with everything on their side but friendship, fall deep into sorrow, struggling to enjoy their childhoods because belonging and connection were never found.

The Friendship Blueprint results from almost 30 years of practice-based evidence involving over 75,000 children across a broad range of neurotypes. Connecting with others has proven time and again to be not just a nice-to-have, but an essential ingredient for social-emotional well-being, purpose, and pro-social behaviour. In a world that can sometimes feel hurried, uncertain, or even a little lonely, the power of friendship is more important than ever. I wrote these pages from my heart, hoping to offer you a blueprint that is both practical and deeply compassionate, a resource you can return to as you support the children in your care and perhaps even as you nurture your own relationships.

When social-emotional well-being is placed at the heart of education. Students not only flourish academically, but also grow into resilient, empathetic, and fulfilled individuals. The evidence is clear: when schools and families prioritise kindness and inclusion, everyone thrives.

As you read, I invite you to reflect on your own story. Who were the friends, mentors, or teachers who helped shape your life? What legacies of kindness and connection do you want to leave for the young people in your care? This book is not just my story, it's ours. The lessons, ideas, and practical tools within are meant to be adapted, shared, and brought to life in ways that honour your unique context and community.

Ultimately, *The Friendship Blueprint* is about hope. It is about believing in the power of connection, even in uncertain times. It is about recognising that each of us, through small acts of kindness, inclusion, and courage, can create ripples that last a lifetime. I am deeply grateful to the children, families, and colleagues who have taught me what true friendship looks like, and to you, the reader, for carrying this legacy forward.

May these pages inspire you to nurture the friendships that will shape not only the lives of children, but also the future of our schools, families, and communities.

With my very best wishes, always, Madhavi

A wish for children around the world, by Ms Lauren Brooks, Principal, St Ignatius' College, SA, December 2025

My wish for young people is a childhood filled with wonder and belonging.

A childhood marked by curiosity, mess, play, exploring, and belly laughs.

A childhood nurtured by adults who love and guide them, and one that is enriched by friendships—the joyful ones that make life bright.

May their formative years be rich with defining moments that teach them how to repair, forgive, and grow.

I wish for them the courage to do hard things, to connect deeply and disconnect wisely, to move through the world with a slow, intentional spirit that ponders interiorly, pays attention to what matters, and finds the good in all things.

And in this landmark moment of bold social-media reform, I wish for them a future where technology serves their humanity, not diminishes it—where their friendships are not reduced to screens but strengthened by presence and compassion.

May our children be shaped by the kind of love that helps them discover who they are, and who they are becoming.

May "The Friendship Blueprint" bring all of this and more to our young people in schools around the world.

Acknowledgements

Sincere thanks to Routledge London and Taylor & Francis Australia for being such wonderful publishers. Thank you to Vilija Stephens and Alison Foyle for believing in this book right from the start. Thank you, Steven Heath, Charlotte Waters, Khadijah Ebrahim, Clare Midgley, Imran Mirza and Sarah Davey for your fantastic communication and generosity with your time and support throughout.

Anne Dunstan, thank you for writing my foreword with such deep care and thought. I'm truly blessed to know you both as a mentor and a friend. You are a gift to education, and I learn so much from you every time we speak. Lauren Brooks, when we first spoke, my heart leapt out of my chest, and I knew you were going to change the world somehow. I couldn't have begun to anticipate how quickly you would do that in such a short time, yet here you are. Thank you for taking the time in your very busy schedule to write a poetic wish for children and friendships. Emma McKenzie, you are an exceptional counsellor, friend and educator, whose work has inspired me for years. What an honour to have your review on my back cover. David Kolpak, for over two decades, we've shared many career milestones. Our conversations are honest and enlightening, and I'm so grateful for our work together and our friendship. Emily Rogers, we have a shared passion and purpose for this topic. You have compassionately led so many young people through the ups and downs of friendship, and it means so much to me that you were so willing to review *The Friendship Blueprint*. Dr Lee Del Col, your genuine, steady effort to connect with and value your students inspires young people to seek connection with and value each other. You have always understood the power of connection and I thank you for reviewing this book. Last but not least, Sarah Shoobridge, thank you. Your willingness to take such deep dives into all things well-being in Education, whether it's for students, educators, or early career teachers, is nothing short of inspirational. Sarah Sutter, thank you for your faith, confidence and generous leadership. Your contribution has been profound, yet delivered with perfect humility. Thank you.

Rachel Reiter, thank you for listening so deeply and taking the time to truly understand what this book is all about. You poured your heart into the front cover and posters, and I can't wait to see them out in the world. Juliette Priestly, thank you for formatting my manuscript so beautifully and enthusiastically. Your genuine care and attention to detail over the final month of manuscript preparation allowed me to take a breath and prepare for the next stage of production. Tom Venus, thank you for your reliable, steady support with the QR code and branding detail. Your willingness to help and genuine desire to do things well will take you far in life, young man.

My heartfelt gratitude to the children and families at Positive Minds Australia who teach me and our PMA Dream Team what the world truly needs, giving us the inspiration to keep playing our part to make the world a better place. Your presence in our work has brought a deeper meaning and purpose into all our lives, and we are forever grateful for the honour you have bestowed upon us, to be the people that help you through your tough times, thank you.

PMA dream team, thank you for working with such authenticity, intelligence, and genuine kindness every day. I love the excitement we burst into when we see each other and the ripple effect that has on our clients every day. You're such a blessing to me and every family you support. Thank you for joining me for the ride.

To my incredible family and friends, who fill my cup every day with limitless love, loyalty, encouragement, wisdom, kindness, and joy, I start every day thankful to each one of you. How did I get so lucky to have you in my life, to learn from and laugh with? Lucky me. 5.30 am club, thank you for starting the day strong with me. Our morning banter often brings a smile to my day, long after the versa has cooled down. GR8 K8 Bolton, thank you for always interrupting me back, and for knowing just what I needed, when I needed it. To James, Soraya, Toby, and Zach, you are more to me than I ever imagined possible. Your presence makes my heart skip a beat every time, even after all these years. Thank you.

To the hard-working educators, parents, researchers, youth workers, allied health, and health professionals, out there humbly doing their part to find answers, to advocate, support, make things better, thank you for everything you've taught me. The world is so much better, thanks to you.

Finally, to all the parents everywhere. You are the most important person in a young person's life. As your child's life unfolds before you, I hope you will always show yourself self-compassion, appreciation for all the sacrifices you make each day, and make time for yourself, even if it's just for a moment.

Introduction

After three decades in psychology and education, I'm proud to share my most passionate work: a blueprint for empowering young people with essential skills to connect with others, experience belonging, and foster compassion, for themselves and those around them.

Over the years, I've seen how quickly a person's wellbeing and personal growth can be hindered by social pain that ends in a broken relationship (Bukowski et al., 2018). Children flourish when they feel seen, heard, and valued by adults and peers (Denham et al., 2003). Valuing every child based on their humanity, character and effort increases their potential and supports their social and emotional wellbeing and opportunity to thrive.

Thousands of young people have told me they never believed belonging was possible (Astington & Jenkins, 1995). Many felt misunderstood for social missteps rooted in their unique wiring, facing isolation and bullying with little patience from those around them (Bukowski et al., 2018). For some, school was their only refuge. A place where dedicated educators offered kindness, stability, and hope, even when resources were stretched thin. These educators are true heroes, inspiring me with their resilience and their unwavering belief in every child's potential.

Happy endings aren't guaranteed, and many challenges are beyond our control (Gifford-Smith & Brownell, 2003). But one caring adult can make a world of difference (Denham et al., 2003). My team and I focus on helping students see their strengths, not just their struggles, offering connection, optimism, and the reminder that their lives truly matter.

Most importantly, we empower parents, caregivers, and teachers with the knowledge, courage, and hope to do their best, and to embrace both their efforts and their imperfections along the way (Collaborative for Academic, Social, and Emotional Learning [CASEL], 2020).

I've witnessed countless young people transform, finding confidence, self-awareness, and hope as they overcome loneliness and discover authentic connection. The evidence is clear: when schools prioritise cultures of kindness and inclusion, using a shared language of connection between students, educators and parents, deep, sustainable change becomes possible (Durlak et al., 2011; Prothero, 2025). Educators can change lives by prioritising warm, meaningful connections, one student at a time.

Imagine a school where every child is equipped for friendship, kindness, compassion and communication. Picture students brimming with courage and empathy, supported by adults who believe in their limitless potential. Social-emotional well-being deserves a place at the heart of our curriculum, on par with literacy and science, because our ability to connect with others is one of the most powerful predictors of life-long happiness and success (CASEL, 2020; Cipriano & Christina, 2023; Durlak et al., 2011).

Shaped by the voices of young people across Australia, this book addresses real-world questions about friendship and belonging in our ever-changing world (Astington & Jenkins, 1995; Bukowski et al., 2018).

Ideal for pre-school to year 8, and easily adaptable for all school ages, The Friendship Blueprint is packed with practical activities frameworks and advice to tackle challenges like miscommunication, emotional struggles, and unkind behaviour (Denham et al., 2003; Gifford-Smith & Brownell, 2003).

Strength-based and evidence-informed, The Friendship Blueprint helps build a culture where differences in neurotypes, learning and communication styles, character, values and social expression are understood to be natural. Throughout the book, students learn how to manage this in a respectful and compassionate way, offering accessible skills rooted in real experiences and genuine inclusion, not in changing who anyone is (CASEL, 2020).

In a world where face-to-face connection is fading, the greatest gift we can give children is skills, opportunities, and practice to experience real time connection where they can experience the profound joy of belonging (Hill et al., 2016).

COVID-related isolation has further affected children's mental health, disrupting crucial stages of social-emotional development (Denham et al., 2003; Doan et al., 2023). Young children lost vital face-to-face experiences, leading to heightened anxiety, behavioural challenges, and disrupted well-being (Centre for Community Child Health, 2022; Easthope, 2022).

The Friendship Blueprint was written against the backdrop of new and evolving challenges. Children today face a "happiness recession," struggling with basic social skills and uncertainty in the wake of the pandemic (Doan et al., 2023; McLaughlin, 2025). Teachers see the impact in every classroom, from difficulty sharing to reluctance to participate. Imagine what's possible when social knowledge and emotional intelligence curriculums like The Friendship Blueprint become the response and solution to turning this around (Astington & Jenkins, 1995).

Uncertainty, increased screen time, and anxiety now affect millions of children and many struggle to meet developmental milestones or attend school regularly (Easthope, 2022; Hill et al., 2016). Our young people need social-emotional skills more than ever (Durlak et al., 2011). They need our support, our creativity, and most of all, our belief in their capacity for connection and growth.

While the long term impact of social media and excessive device use on developing brains is still emerging (Hill et al., 2016). We do know that these influences disrupt communication and self-regulation skills (Denham et al., 2003). Building student capacity in social emotional knowledge and skills, is a powerful and proactive step towards protecting their future.

The Friendship Blueprint empowers all students to safely, confidently and uniquely contribute with pride, to the social fabric (Bukowski et al., 2018). When young people feel they belong, they can flourish; socially, emotionally, and academically (Denham et al., 2003; Durlak et al., 2011).

Evidence-informed

The Friendship Blueprint is a structured, evidence-informed framework to build student capacity in social-emotional learning (SEL). Research by Collaborative for Academic, Social, and Emotional Learning (CASEL, 2020), Selman (1980), Gifford-Smith and Brownell (2003), and Bukowski et al. (2018) evidence based Core Friendship Skills Model, below, is carefully considered and included throughout The Friendship Blueprint lesson plans.

1. ***Self-Awareness (understanding your own emotions and social role)***
   Understanding our emotions and being self-aware is crucial for understanding universal social knowledge and realising our social role. Belonging and connection is essential for social-emotional well-being. Social roles in our communities differ for everyone, but kindness, psychological safety, and respect for our fellow humans are common threads we can all endeavour to uphold. Our social role can be as simple as being genuine and kind, or it can be celebrating our own and other people's diversity and welcoming neurodivergent and neurotypical thinking equally, or it might be to hold a peaceful nature that provides steadiness in the chaos. When self-awareness is strong, a steady culture of warmth, compassion, and connection can thrive.

2. ***Communication skills (verbal and non-verbal interaction)***
   Safe and friendly communication, openness and warmth, noticing and welcoming others, active and reflective listening, kindness, and empathy all mean something different to each of us and are by no means intended as essential skills for experiencing social success. Some cultures and neurodivergent people find some verbal and non-verbal communication approaches unnatural, undesirable, unnecessary, unhelpful, and even distressing. Respecting this and helping all students and educators understand cultural differences and neurodivergence creates inclusive, aware, and welcoming environments despite differences in verbal and non-verbal communication styles.

   Accurately interpreting and applying verbal and non-verbal communication skills often makes social interactions easier, and learning them can reduce anxiety and increase confidence. Students can all grow together in understanding and awareness of different social interaction preferences, and then commit to doing their best to be kind, gentle, and respectful communicators.

3. ***Empathy and perspective taking (Understanding others' feelings)***
   Many social challenges children face occur because their ability to see things from other people's perspectives, put themselves in other children's shoes, and empathise is still in the early stages of development. Some young people haven't had these important skills modelled to them and struggle to offer them to others. Most young people just need time and

guidance to develop and strengthen this valuable skill for healthy relationships. Noticing other people's emotions and perspectives, and responding with kindness, takes time and practice, but once it's there, it connects us to the most pleasant neurotransmitters, like serotonin and oxytocin, which are released when we are in deep connection with another person's feelings.

4. ***Conflict resolution and problem solving (Handling disagreements positively)***

   Conflict in childhood and adolescence is a sign of a strong, healthy brain navigating the social landscape while developing self-awareness and social awareness within an unpredictable, sometimes highly reactive emotional system. Social clumsiness, inexperience, and emotional immaturity provide the perfect storm. Learning to pause, reflect, consider the other person, and, where appropriate, compromise and negotiate in conflict are hard enough skills for adults, and it's important to be realistic when expecting this from children. As children's brains remain emotionally underdeveloped and unpredictable until their mid to late 20s, it's only reasonable that we teach with compassion and understanding, without expecting unrealistic outcomes.

5. ***Inclusion and cooperation (Building and maintaining friendships)***

   Understanding the how and why of inclusion and cooperation brings young people confidence to connect in a kind and pro-social manner. Encouraging students to work together and practice collaborative play gives them a head start when handling challenging situations where emotions run high. Understanding bias and exclusion, as well as neurodivergence and culture, is crucial for enhancing the depth, authenticity, and sustainability of social relationships.

This Core Friendship Skills Model is based on research showing how whole school SEL initiatives help create agency and self confidence through

Figure 0.1 QR code link to social media

crucial human centred skill acquisition that can improve peer relationships, emotional regulation, and academic outcomes (Durlak et al., 2011). By explicitly teaching these five areas throughout "The Friendship Blueprint," provides a strong foundation to influence lifelong social-emotional well-being and healthy relationship skills.

Every student, class and culture is unique. Your confidence to tailor this curriculum to who you're teaching using your personal and professional knowledge and experience, will profoundly impact how it sticks and stays in a young person's mind in the years to come. To enhance your skills and knowledge, please join me on Instagram, Facebook, and TikTok.

Here's to you and all that's ahead.

Curriculum connections

The Friendship Blueprint directly meets key criteria of the Australian Health and Well-being Curriculum and is relevant for schools globally. It provides practical strategies and knowledge to help teachers create an environment where all students have a better chance to develop friendships, and actively and pro socially participate in their communities.

Chapter 1 strongly aligns with the Australian Curriculum for Health and Physical Education, focusing on personal, social, and emotional well-being. Through activities and reflections, students develop self-awareness, emotional regulation, empathy, and respectful relationships. They learn to express emotions, build strengths, communicate positively, and resolve conflict, directly meeting content descriptors. This evidence-based approach builds crucial capabilities for lifelong health, well-being, and positive social interactions.

Chapter 2 closely aligns with the Australian Curriculum's health and social-emotional well-being requirements. It explicitly teaches self-awareness, emotional regulation, empathy, communication, and conflict resolution through evidence-based practices. Activities such as reflective discussions, role-plays, and problem-solving build self-management, social awareness, and relationship skills, meeting key curriculum criteria. This ensures students gain essential social and emotional skills for well-being and lifelong learning.

Chapter 3 aligns with the Australian Curriculum's health and social-emotional well-being requirements. Students learn to manage emotions, understand the effects of overthinking, and develop self-awareness. Activities focus on communication, empathy, perspective-taking, and conflict resolution, supporting respectful relationships and emotional literacy. The chapter promotes resilience, inclusion, and adaptability, fulfilling curriculum goals for social and emotional well-being and positive relationship skills.

Chapter 4 explicitly develops students' personal and social capability, as outlined in the Australian Curriculum. Structured activities build self-awareness, social awareness, communication, and relationship skills. The traffic light model offers practical tools for navigating friendships, fostering healthy relationships, and managing peer challenges, directly supporting curriculum criteria for well-being.

Chapter 5 meets the Australian Curriculum's requirements for health and social-emotional well-being, with a focus on Personal and Social Capability and Health and Physical Education. Through evidence-based activities, students develop self-awareness, emotional regulation, empathy, respectful relationships, and communication skills. The chapter also addresses diversity, neurodivergence, and inclusion, reflecting curriculum priorities for well-being and positive school communities.

Chapter 6 aligns with the Health and Physical Education strand and the Personal and Social Capability requirements of the Australian Curriculum. Students build self-awareness, empathy, communication, and conflict resolution skills through group discussions, self-reflection, role-plays, and kindness initiatives. These activities help students develop positive relationships, emotional regulation, and inclusive, respectful interactions, supporting key curriculum outcomes for health and well-being.

Chapter 7 delivers on the Australian Curriculum's requirements for health and social-emotional well-being. Students practise core Personal and Social Capability skills—managing emotions, developing empathy, building respectful relationships, making responsible decisions, and resolving conflict. Lessons use reflection, role-play, restorative conversations, and games to teach communication, boundary-setting, and problem-solving strategies, equipping young people to manage relationships and build resilience.

Chapter 8 meets the Australian Curriculum's Health and Physical Education and Personal and Social Capability requirements. Through activities and reflections, students develop self-awareness, resilience, and respectful relationships. The chapter emphasises psychological safety, diversity, empathy, conflict resolution, and communication skills, fostering inclusive, supportive communities and preparing students to contribute positively to their health and well-being.

Chapter 9 closely aligns with Australian Curriculum requirements in health and social-emotional well-being. Students learn self-awareness, self-management, social awareness, and social management through evidence-based activities. The chapter teaches students to recognise healthy friendships, set boundaries, resolve conflicts, and communicate empathetically, promoting inclusion, resilience, and positive peer relationships both offline and online.

The difference between evidence informed and evidence based.
The Friendship Blueprint is an evidence informed framework grounded in contemporary educational and neurodevelopmental research, while also drawing on almost 30 years providing training and support to thousands of educators, families and allied health professionals across Australia. While evidence based programs are validated through formal research studies under controlled conditions, evidence informed programs go a step further by integrating the best available research with clinical expertise, practitioner insight and real-world application. Published through Routledge following rigorous international peer review, The Friendship Blueprint offers schools a scientifically credible, practical and highly implementable framework for strengthening friendship skills, emotional wellbeing and positive school culture."The Friendship Blueprint" is the book I needed as a child, and knew I had to write as an adult. Inside, you'll find a practical, evidence-informed toolkit that can easily be tailored to teach foundational skills for friendliness that enable more regulated, self aware and socially aware capabilities in students that easily translate to real life (Bukowski et al., 2018; CASEL, 2020; Durlak et al., 2011). These strategies empower young people to better understand how to connect, communicate, and create communities where everyone belongs.

References

Astington, J. W., & Jenkins, J. M. (1995). Theory of mind development and social understanding. *Cognitive Development, 10*(1), 39–62.

Bukowski, W. M., Laursen, B., & Rubin, K. H. (2018). *Handbook of peer interactions, relationships, and groups*. Guilford Press.

Centre for Community Child Health. (2022). Rapid review prepared by the Centre for Community Child Health, Murdoch Children's Research Institute for the Commonwealth Department of Education, Skills and Employment.

Cipriano, & Christina. (2023). Research finds social and emotional learning produces significant benefits for students. *Child Development 94*. https://medicine.yale.edu/news-article/new-research-published-in-child-development-confirms-social-and-emotional-learning-significantly-improves-student-academic-performance-well-being-and-perceptions-of-school-safety/

Collaborative for Academic, Social, and Emotional Learning (CASEL). (2020). SEL competencies framework. https://casel.org/

Denham, S. A., Blair, K. A., DeMulder, E., Levitas, J., Sawyer, K., Auerbach–Major, S., & Queenan, P. (2003). Social-emotional learning in early childhood. *Early Education & Development, 14*(1), 101–119.

Doan, S. N., Burniston, A. B., Smiley, P., & Liu, C. H. (2023). COVID-19 pandemic and changes in children's behavioral problems: The mediating role of maternal depressive symptoms. *Children, 10*(6), 977. https://doi.org/10.3390/children10060977

Durlak, J. A., Weissberg, R. P., Dymnicki, A. B., Taylor, R. D., & Schellinger, K. B. (2011). The impact of enhancing students' social and emotional learning: A meta-analysis of school-based universal interventions. *Child Development 82*(1), 405–432. https://doi.org/10.1111/j.1467-8624.2010.01564.x

Easthope, L. (2022). When the dust settles: Stories of love, loss and hope from an expert in disaster. *Hodder & Stoughton*. https://www.hodder.co.uk/titles/lucy-easthope/when-the-dust-settles/9781529384260/

Gifford-Smith, M. E., & Brownell, C. A. (2003). Childhood peer relationships. *Journal of School Psychology, 41*(4), 235–284.

Hill, D., Ameenuddin, N., Chassiakos, Y. R., Cross, C., Hutchinson, J., Levine, A., Boyd, R., Mendelson, R., Moreno, M., & Swanson, W. S. (2016). Media and young minds. *Pediatrics, 138*(5). https://doi.org/10.1542/peds.2016-2591

McLaughlin, C. (2025). Children's Laureate Cottrell-Boyce warns early years reading at 'crisis point'. https://www.standard.co.uk/showbiz/celebrity-news/government-keir-starmer-cressida-cowell-bridget-phillipson-steve-rotheram-b1206258.html

Prothero, A. (2025). Social-emotional learning linked to higher math and reading test scores. *Education Week, 45*. https://www.edweek.org/leadership/social-emotional-learning-linked-to-higher-math-and-reading-test-scores/2025/10

Selman, R. L. (1980). *The growth of interpersonal understanding: Developmental and clinical analyses*. Academic Press.

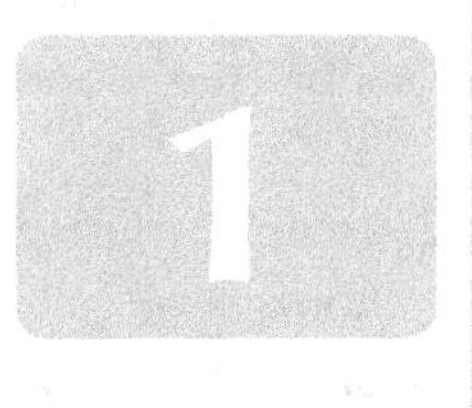

How friendship strengthens our social-emotional well-being

While we know friendship is central to happiness and wellbeing, friendly school cultures don't just happen; they grow from a shared language of kindness, compassion and inclusion with a deliberate plan for pro-social skill development

Learning quest

Friendships are vital for well-being, bringing safety, connection, and purpose. As social beings, we're hardwired to belong to a group, which helps us thrive (Selman, 1997). Even one supportive friend can make a profound difference in a child's life, showing them they are seen and valued. This chapter helps children recognise how friendships boost confidence, happiness, and well-being.

Setting the scene

Decades of research show that strong friendships are closely linked to better mental health and happiness (Güroğlu, 2022; Selman, 1997). Meaningful connections build trust and empathy and reduce loneliness, anxiety, and depression (Erol & Köksal, 2025).

Spending time with friends releases neurotransmitters like dopamine and oxytocin, helping us cope with challenges, build confidence, and enjoy school.

DOI: 10.4324/9781003617570-1

Healthy friendships bring joy and a sense of unity, while negative friendships can leave us feeling insecure and lonely. As Woodrow Wilson once pointed out, "friendship is the only cement that will ever hold the world together."

Good friendships fuel well-being, boost happiness, and protect us during tough times.

Friendships encourage positive actions and foster personal growth by offering new perspectives.

Even as digital interactions increase, real friendships create authentic bonds that reduce loneliness and offer support. Strong social-emotional well-being makes learning and managing emotions easier.

Spotting the skills in action

Shreya and Max's stories show how friendship challenges and successes affect well-being, highlighting the difference between strong and weak friendships (Self-Awareness, Empathy, Perspective Taking).

Shreya's surprise

Shreya was one of the kindest people you could meet. She loved animals, her friends, her family, and could do the splits, then leap into a cartwheel with ease. Shreya loved her birthday and spent all her pocket money to make it special. For her, birthdays were a time to thank and spoil the people she loved.

On the day Shreya carried her birthday invitations, she bounced with excitement, grinned widely, and couldn't wait to hand them out. As she entered the yard, her friends ran off, laughing and holding hands. Shreya didn't know why, and for the first time, she felt a sinking feeling in her stomach.

The day only got worse. Shreya's invitations sat in her school bag, weighed down by whispers and laughs whenever she looked up. The sick feeling in her stomach grew. When students paired up for a project, everyone except Shreya got chosen. No one turned to include her. Tears came to her eyes. It felt like the worst day she'd ever had. She could hardly breathe, standing alone while everyone else chatted. Things got worse when she overheard plans for a slumber party on the weekend she was planning her own. Shreya's tears flowed faster, and her embarrassment burned her cheeks. She wanted to go home, and it wasn't even recess. The bell rang, and her friends ran outside without her; she ate recess alone.

Day after day, she got the same cold response, with no explanation. Shreya begged her parents to let her change schools; she couldn't bear it. She lay awake every night, dreading the next day. Her body stayed tense, she got sick more often, and happiness felt impossible. One morning, Shreya couldn't get out of bed. Her sadness was heavy, and she was exhausted. This lasted for months. No one from school visited except her teacher. Shreya didn't see the point in going back. She had fallen far behind in class, and no one knew how to help. The Shreya everyone knew was a shadow of herself.

Student reflection

How was Shreya feeling when she arrived at school with her party invitations?

How do you know how she was feeling?

Why do you think what happened made her mood feel terrible so quickly?

Why do you think her friends changed how they treated her all of a sudden, without any warning?

What would you do if you were Shreya?

What would you do if you were a teacher at the school?

Would you want someone to step in and help if this happened to you?

Max's story

Max loved basketball. He played for his school and club, and had a great last season. At club trials, he and his friends walked in, nervous but excited, talking and laughing. His club teammates were also his best friends; some of them went to school with him.

After a few weeks, the new club teams were announced. Max was in a great mood, he'd just been named school captain. As names were called, the boys high-fived each other. The coach finished, but Max's name was left out. The coach gave him a sympathetic look. Max felt a lump in his throat. His hands, pressed into his legs, had gone white.

Max had never faced such disappointment. He got home, shut his door, and cried. He skipped dinner. When he was about to scream, his friends knocked on his door. One jumped on his bed and acted silly, making Max laugh. Another brought snacks and asked, "Are you coming with us?" The others had basketballs. Max's mum told him to go to the park, hinting there would be no TV if he didn't. He went with a small smile. No one mentioned basketball; they just played and had fun. On the way home, Max brought up the trials. Everyone said they were surprised and that the game would not be the same without him. Eliza said she felt bad for Martin, who had never been chosen. Max realised others had also received bad news. He remembered his dad teaching him that setbacks are part of life. When tough times come, it's better to ask, "Why not me?" Max felt better as soon as his friends arrived. After the game, he felt like himself again. Now, everything seemed okay.

Max slept well that night. The next day at school, he thanked his friends for helping him and tried to see himself in Martin and in all the others who didn't make it. He even went to watch the first club game of the season.

Student reflection:
What did you learn from Max's story?
What kind of person do you think Max is?
How did he get out of his mood so quickly?
What do you think Max's Dad meant by, "Instead of why me, why not me?"

Thank your students for listening during the story, invite them to close their eyes, and ask them to take a moment to imagine themselves in Shreya's position, then in Max's. This moment allows for empathy to be further extended, providing another step towards deeper empathy and compassion, the foundation for deep, meaningful friendships. (Empathy and Perspective Taking)

Friendship web

Have students sit in a circle with a ball of yarn. Turn this into a game by using different coloured yarns for different types of support (kindness, helping, cheering up, etc.), so the web becomes colourful, and students can see the variety of ways friends help each other. Add a "mystery friend" twist: after sharing, students try to guess who tossed them the yarn or recall a specific act of kindness they've seen in the class. This keeps everyone engaged and deepens their attention to classmates' actions. Wrap up with a group challenge: can they untangle the web together without letting go of their yarn? This fosters teamwork and a sense of fun while reinforcing the lesson. Ask your students, "How do these connections help us when challenges come up? What would happen if someone dropped their thread?" Encourage reflection on how each person's support strengthens the group and helps everyone thrive.

Educator reflection. (Self-Awareness, Empathy, and Perspective Taking)

When have you noticed a child struggle with their social-emotional well-being?

How have you known they are struggling?

What do you usually look for in children to check in on their social-emotional well-being? (i.e., how do you know they are okay/not okay?)

How do you check in with children to assess the health and well-being of their social-emotional lives?

How healthy and positive do you feel the relational dynamics of your class/family are most of the time?

What have you learnt about the power of friendships for social-emotional well-being from this chapter so far?

What would you add from your knowledge and experience?

You know yourself better than anyone else, or do you? (Self-Awareness)

Self-awareness is essential for learning and growth. Without self-awareness, it's very difficult for a child or an adult to learn from their mistakes and continue on the path towards becoming the best version of themselves. Turning inward, being honest with yourself to identify your strengths and weaknesses, accepting constructive feedback, and being accountable for your mistakes can be extremely uncomfortable for even the most self-aware person.

Before inviting your students to do this, take a moment to reflect on yourself and identify areas where you know you can improve in your relationships. Usually, there's something we can do better, whether it's making more effort to reach out and check in on loved ones, avoiding gossip, or choosing family and friends over work. Think about why it's hard for you to prioritise working on this and what the negative consequences might be if you don't make a change.

Invite your students to stretch out and take a seat on the floor. Please let them know that they may feel a little uncomfortable and vulnerable during this exercise, as many people do. In a notebook, invite them to write or draw about a time that reflects the following three questions: Self-Awareness, Conflict Resolution, and Problem Solving.

1. Think of a time you felt like you didn't belong. What happened, and how did you feel about it? If you can't think of a time this happened to you, count yourself lucky and see if you can think of a time, you saw it happen to another person.
2. Think of a time you wished you had handled a problem with a friend better. What happened?
3. Think of a time you felt proud of the friend you were. What happened?

Reassure students that social mistakes are normal because emotional regulation and perspective-taking develop over many years (Guy-Evans, 2025). Mistakes are part of learning to be a good friend. Remind yourself and your students that no one is expected to be perfect at relationships during childhood or adolescence.

More about me, movie (Communication Skills, Self-Awareness)

Invite each student to reflect on the following questions.

> My favourite challenge.
> My least favourite challenge.
> Something that embarrasses me.
> Something that makes me proud.
> The hardest thing I've ever done.
> The easiest thing I've ever done.
> What I wish I were better at.
> My least favourite feeling of all.
> People I look up to.

Once they've had a chance to write or draw their answers, divide them into groups of three: one person interviews, asking the questions mentioned earlier; another person is being interviewed; and the third person films it. To make it more engaging, allow students to use props or costumes for their "interviews," or create a mock TV show setting. For younger students, you can turn this into a "show and tell" where they introduce their partner using drawings or favourite objects if filming feels too formal. Once all three have been interviewed (with notes in hand is fine), make time to present these to the parents/caregivers and the class over time. (Communication Skills, Empathy, and Perspective Taking)

Knowing me, knowing you, game

In pairs, invite students to stand back-to-back and on "go," turn around toward their partner and express one of three emotions: angry, bored, or happy. For extra fun, have the class brainstorm silly emotions or create their own, like "super excited" or "mystified," and add them to the game. After each round, let students briefly explain why they chose that emotion or share a time they felt that way with a friend. This adds laughter and helps students connect their feelings to real-life situations. Remind the class that no one gets social cues right every time, and that's why kind, respectful communication is key. (Communication Skills, Self-Awareness)

You know your friends, or do you (social awareness)? (Empathy and Perspective Taking, Communication Skills)

When children are very young, they often form friendships with other children who share similar interests. They generally aren't thinking deeply about character and values in pre-school and Junior Primary. Other children's behaviour is often categorised simplistically as "they're nice" or "they're mean," and they might just need one example of kindness or meanness to decide which end of the spectrum they sit on! With a little more experience and time at school, children start to see how they are similar and different from a character and values lens, too. It's much more subtle than it becomes in high school, but there is still a clear shift from "nice" and "mean" to being more specific about the behaviours they like and those that frustrate them.

Taking the time to get to know your friends better and remember details that matter to them helps everyone feel seen, heard, and valued. The trust that grows from this extra effort can strengthen friendships but to do this well, children need to be good listeners. This is the challenging part, particularly with young, developing brains that are often still egocentric, wanting to share their own thoughts and do what they want above all else.

Getting to know you, interviews

Bring students together and divide them into pairs. Offer the following questions (younger students may only be able to answer one at a time), invite students to interview each other, and then have them present to the class about the peer they interviewed. (Communication Skills, Empathy, and Perspective Taking)

Where's your favourite place?

What's your favourite thing to do in your spare time?

If you were a household appliance, which appliance would you be and why?

If you had to wear only one colour for the rest of your life, what colour would you choose?

Encourage students to take notes and drawings to remember their partner's answers. Turn this into a fun memory game: after presentations, quiz the class with playful questions about their peers, awarding small prizes or stickers for correct answers. Give them an extra moment to genuinely review and try remembering these details about them before presenting the interviews to the class. Encourage students to try and remember details about each other and conclude by emphasising the power of wholeheartedly noticing and remembering details about each other, to build trust and closeness. Challenge your students to try and get to know as many people at school as possible, to strengthen their social awareness, empathy, and social knowledge.

Invite each pair to introduce their partner by answering the three questions. Encourage the value of being present and really listening so they, too, learn more about their peers.

The highs and lows of my age (and is it the same for everyone?) *(Empathy and Perspective Taking, Self-Awareness)*

Share how you've been trying to remember what it was like to be their age and how every age has its ups and downs, while everyone is doing their best with the skills and knowledge they have so far. Often, peers are there for all the ups and downs, while going through their own. Let them know that it's hard to remember that everyone wakes up wanting a good day, but at their age, they're still learning to navigate the inevitable social mishaps that come with it.

Hand out construction paper and invite every student to find their own space in the room with markers. The point of the exercise is to write or draw what it feels like to be their age. On one side, they write or draw everything that's great about being their age, and on the other side, they write everything that's hard. They do not write their name on these (make sure they know that right at the start). Ask them to think as hard as they can about the things adults probably don't remember about being that age, so their part in this research can be used to help other children their age.

Once everyone has had a chance to return them to you, give everyone a chance to move and grab a drink of water so they are ready for some role plays.

Make it clear there is no need to guess who wrote the answers when you start exploring them. Use scenarios that are relevant and appropriate to share, that you believe will help open their eyes to other people's experience of being that age. Make sure you focus on both the highs and lows.

Continue on with these until the end of the lesson, finishing each charade with this reflection: Empathy and Perspective Taking, Self-Awareness.

Can you think of a time you felt that way?
Are you surprised that someone your age has these highs and lows?
If you had one of the lows, would you want someone to help you through it?

As you close the lesson, wish them well and support them in remembering: everyone wants a good day, everyone needs friends, and it's hard to know what other people might be struggling with, so always choose kindness.

Win-win solutions because everyone's well-being matters. (Conflict Resolution and Problem Solving, Communication Skills)

Remind them, all around the world, friendship glitches happen, even to the kindest people.

On your whiteboard or butcher's paper, start a brainstorm and ask your students, "What can go wrong in a friendship?" Remind them not to give examples that expose another person's identity. (Conflict Resolution and Problem Solving)

Examples you can add if they aren't covered include:

One person wants to stay friends, but the other person has grown apart.
One friend is being intentionally mean.
One friend will only be friends outside of school and ignore you at school.
One friend always chooses what you do.
A friend puts you down, but you always have fun together when they're kind.

Allow the group to work in pairs, where each person chooses one friendship problem from the brainstorm to solve in a way that's a win-win for both people. To boost engagement, let each pair create a short skit, comic strip, or puppet show to act out their solution. Encourage silly voices or props to make it memorable and fun! A win-win situation is when the people involved in a friendship problem come up with a solution that's fair and acceptable to everyone. Sometimes, one of the friends will need to give up a bit of what they are hoping for, so that everything is fair and kind for all. Allow plenty of time to come up with rich solutions that aren't rushed, and to remember that they never know; their Role-play solution might be helping someone in the class who hasn't spoken out, so what they do matters. Help them see themselves as serving their peers in meaningful, purposeful ways.

Sharing win-win solutions

Return to the circle and ask everyone to share some win-win solutions for friendship problems. Transform the sharing into a "Friendship Fair," where students set up booths or stations to present their win-win solutions through posters, skits, or artwork. Invite other classes or parents to visit and celebrate students' ideas. As a group, create personal posters of their favourite win-win solutions to paste in their notebooks or display in the classroom.

> **Before ending the lesson, take a moment for reflection**
> What's one win-win solution I learned today that I can use?
> What's one friendship problem I've been through that someone else talked about today?
> What's one friendship problem I had no idea some people go through?

Timing matters (self-awareness and social awareness) for everyone's well-being. (Self-Awareness, Communication Skills, Conflict Resolution, and Problem Solving)

There's a time and place for everything. When you're young, timing isn't a priority; it's more about the here and now. This is one of the many reasons why so much can go wrong among children: they often exhibit strong emotions, impulsivity, and egocentricity. The earlier these life skills are taught, the better, for when they are teenagers and adults with bigger decisions to make and more complex relationship dynamics.

When it comes to timing in social situations, self-awareness and social awareness are essential. It's all about being in tune with your own emotions and impulses, while being aware of what someone else is doing or needing, when you want to connect with them or address a challenge with them. (Self-Awareness, Empathy, and Perspective Taking)

Take, for example, two friends who've had a falling out over a group project where the distribution of labour felt uneven. The person who is feeling defensive might want to hash it all out, there and then, while the other person needs time to recover from feeling hurt and doesn't feel like talking at that time. Another situation might be a child, full of excitement, unable to wait until they are alone before handing a birthday invitation to their best friend, then handing it to them in front of other children who aren't invited.

After sharing the two earlier examples (or others that are more relevant to your students), ask your students the following questions and record answers on the whiteboard or butcher paper.

What does "timing" in social situations mean to you?
Can you think of an example of a situation where timing matters in
  a friendship?
How might someone get timing wrong?
How do you know if the timing is right?
How can you make things better if you get the timing wrong?

Their answers have provided plenty of food for thought for role plays. Invite your students to come up with silly and unhelpful examples of timing, especially in the context of resolving conflict with a friend (e.g., chasing them out onto the pitch as they are about to bat in cricket). Have some fun with it and let them have a laugh, gently steering them back on track. There's a time and place for everything. When you're in public, is not the time for private discussions, when you're upset with a friend, don't approach them in front of an audience, when someone is in the middle of something ask them when it's a good time to talk, when a person is upset, give them time to cool down and check they are ready to talk and when a person is trying to focus and concentrate is not the time to distract them with what you could do instead together. (Self-Awareness, Communication Skills, Conflict Resolution, and Problem Solving)

After the role plays, have one last discussion about being "timing aware", especially when they are upset. Teach them how, when emotions run high, thinking runs low. The thinking part of our brains goes offline when feelings are intense, putting us into fight-or-flight or freeze mode, focusing on survival rather than thriving. Trying to solve a problem when we're emotional risks saying or doing something we later regret.

Before finishing the lesson, offer the final reflection questions:
How easy is it for you to use good timing in social situations? What helps it feel easy for you?
How hard is it for you to use good timing in social situations? What makes it hard for you?

Using strengths to improve social-emotional well-being. (Self-Awareness, Empathy, and Perspective Taking)

As we come to the end of this chapter, I'd like to close with the importance of helping students adopt an abundance mindset rather than a deficit mindset when thinking about the people around us.

We're wired with a natural negativity bias, a tendency to notice problems more than positives, to help us stay safe (Norris, 2021). Today, this bias can make us focus on negatives even when there's no real danger.

This can mean we're more likely to notice what we don't like about someone more quickly than what we do. We do this to ourselves too, focusing on what we don't like about our faces, hair, bodies, and personalities, rather than all the aspects that are right about them.

Before we can truly open our hearts to the good in others, we must first seek it out within ourselves. Knowing what's good and right about us is essential, and oftentimes this comes from our caregivers and educators who complemented and supported our strengths. For some, their caregivers focused more on their weaknesses, which can make it hard for them to feel confident in themselves.

Everyone has unique strengths. Recognising and using them builds confidence and helps us appreciate others' strengths. Focusing on strengths, rather than weaknesses, supports social-emotional well-being.

Using our strengths in relationships makes us feel confident and energised. Practising this habit, looking for what's good in ourselves and others, builds social awareness, compassion, and kindness.

Allow your students some reflection time to think about what they feel their personal strengths might be, and as you walk around the room, let each student know a strength you've noticed in them. If your students are 8 or older, they can take a survey like viacharacter.org. (Self-Awareness)

Using strengths to uplift others and spread social-emotional well-being (Empathy and Perspective Taking)

Write your students' names on a Paddle Pop stick and add them to a jar. In a moment, they will have the opportunity to draw a name from the jar. Their job is to utilise their strengths and best qualities to serve as a gentle mentor to that person. The trick is that the person can't know you're their mentor. The student's role is to be a subtle but steady and helpful presence for the person they have been randomly assigned to. Remind them how everyone wakes up in the morning wanting to have a good day. How things unfold between peers during the day can have the biggest impact of all on how a person feels about their day at the end of it. This activity is one small way to tighten the social thread.

Each week, allow students to choose someone new to keep it novel. For added excitement, host a "Secret Strengths Celebration" at the end of each month, where students guess who their secret mentor was and share stories about acts of kindness they received. Watch the warmth and connection grow as the culture of mentorship, peer support, and kindness evolves.

Key takeaways: Chapter 1: How friendship strengthens our social-emotional well-being

- **Friendship is fundamental:** Strong friendships are essential for children's happiness and sense of belonging (Güroğlu, 2022).

- **Well-being boost:** Supportive friendships help children manage challenges and grow emotionally. Even one caring friend makes a real difference (Erol & Köksal, 2025).
- **Emotional impact:** Healthy friendships boost mood and resilience; negative ones can lead to loneliness.
- **Skills for life: Building and repairing** friendships teaches kindness, empathy, and conflict resolution.
- **Self and social awareness:** Understanding one's own feelings, strengths, and challenges, and appreciating others' perspectives, is crucial for fostering healthy friendships and promoting social-emotional growth.
- **Empathy and inclusion:** Practising empathy, noticing when others struggle, and choosing to be kind or inclusive strengthens both individuals and the group.
- **Handling ups and downs:** Everyone experiences challenges in friendships. Learning when and how to communicate, and reflecting on timing in social situations, helps solve problems constructively.
- **Strengths-based approach:** Focusing on personal and others' strengths builds confidence and creates a positive, supportive environment for all.
- **Community matters:** A culture that values and nurtures friendship supports emotional resilience, not just for individuals, but for the whole group or classroom.

Call to action

Let's create a culture where friendships aren't just encouraged, they're intentionally nurtured as a core part of every student's growth. Use this chapter to spark conversations, build connection-rich environments, and empower students to understand the vital role friendships play in their emotional resilience and sense of belonging. Remind them that emotional resilience comes from how the group and community work together, not from individual responsibility alone.

Embed friendship-focused language into classroom routines, celebrate acts of kindness and empathy, and provide regular opportunities for students to reflect on how friendships impact their feelings, choices, and sense of identity. Assign class "Friendship Ambassadors" to lead weekly check-ins and brainstorm ways to welcome new students or support classmates who may feel left out. Encourage students to develop and vote on a class friendship charter that outlines shared values and practical commitments.

Encourage staff to model healthy relationship-building and create safe spaces where students feel seen, supported, and valued. Share success stories of friendship and inclusion in assemblies or newsletters to inspire the whole community. When friendship becomes the foundation of school life, students thrive—not only socially but also emotionally and academically.

Together, let's make friendship a strength that supports the well-being of every learner. Set a clear action plan: make friendship a daily priority, celebrate acts of kindness, model healthy relationship skills, and create regular opportunities for reflection and connection. Encourage students to set weekly friendship goals, such as reaching out to someone new or practising a win-win approach, and to reflect on their progress at the end of each week. Provide a class display or journal for recording moments of friendship and growth, so students can see the positive impact over time.

References

Erol, M., & Köksal, H. (2025). The effect of friendship education on primary school students' psychological well-being and peer relationships. *Child Indicators Research, 18*. https://doi.org/10.1007/s12187-025-10221-1

Güroğlu, B. (2022). The power of friendship: The developmental significance of friendships from a neuroscience perspective. *Child Development Perspectives, 16*(2), 110–117. https://doi.org/10.1111/cdep.12450

Guy-Evans, O. (2025). When does the prefrontal cortex fully develop? *Simply Psychology*. https://www.simplypsychology.org/prefrontal-cortex-development-age.html

Norris, C. (2021). The negativity bias, revisited: Evidence from neuroscience measures and an individual differences approach. *Social Neuroscience, 16*, 1–15. https://pubmed.ncbi.nlm.nih.gov/31750790/

Selman, R. L. (1997). *Fostering friendship: Pair therapy for treatment and prevention*. Harvard University Press. https://www.hup.harvard.edu/catalog.php?isbn=9780674000190

Appendix: Practical Tools and Tips

Quick Reference Table – Friendship Activities

Activity Name	Age Group	Materials Needed	Key Learning Goals

| Friendship Web | Primary | Yarn (various colours) | Connection, teamwork, empathy |

| Interview Game/Show & Tell | Primary | Paper, pens, props/costumes | Listening, empathy, self-awareness |

| Emotion Game | Primary | None | Communication, emotional literacy |

| Win-Win Skits & Fair | Primary | Paper, markers, props | Conflict resolution, creativity |

| Secret Strengths Celebration | Primary | Paddle pop sticks, jar | Kindness, mentoring |

Teacher tips and troubleshooting

Have flexible roles for shy students. Let them observe or choose a helper buddy.
Use visuals and drawing alternatives for students who prefer or need
    non-verbal communication.
If a group is restless, switch to a movement-based activity or break large
    tasks into bite-sized steps.

Student self-reflection/assessment

"How did I help a friend this week?"
"What is one friendship skill I want to practice next week?"
"What is one thing I noticed about someone else's strengths?"

Teacher reflection prompts

What worked well in these activities?
Which strategies helped include every learner?
What will I adapt for next time?

Family and community links

Send home a "Friendship Conversation Starter" slip: "Ask someone at home
    about a time friendship helped them."
Invite families to contribute to a class "friendship mural" or share stories.
Feature student friendship stories in the school newsletter.

Inclusion and accessibility reminders

Adapt activities for all learners: allow choices between drawing, writing, speaking, or acting.
Pair students thoughtfully and rotate partners to build new bonds.
Have a quiet space available for students who feel overwhelmed.

Real-life stories and scenarios

Use short, relatable vignettes (see Shreya and Max's stories) to spark discussion.
Share anonymised student quotes: "Friendship is… helping me when I'm sad."

Ongoing practice

Make friendship skills part of weekly routines. Try "Friendship Fridays" or a rotating "Friendship Leader."
Revisit activities each term and celebrate progress.

Why it works: The research

Every activity in this chapter is based on research showing that social-emotional skills, especially friendship-building, are linked to well-being, academic success, and inclusion (see References for details).
Strong classroom relationships reduce bullying, foster empathy, and help every student feel they belong.
These tools are designed to make friendship learning practical and lasting for every reader, educator, and student.

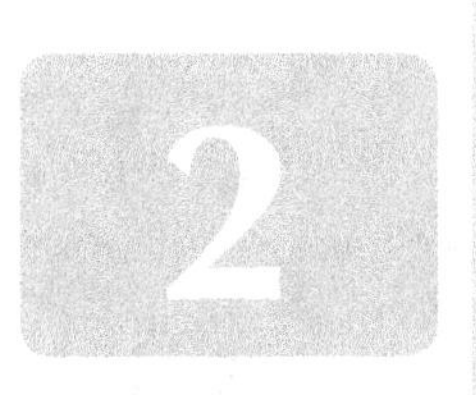

How emotional regulation helps friendships

When entering the classroom, a child's central nervous system immediately tunes into the emotional regulation state of peers and educators. Connection is less likely to happen when theirs or other people's dysregulated emotions are in the driver's seat.

Learning quest (Self-Awareness, Emotional Regulation)

Imagine your feelings as superpowers! When you're angry, frustrated, jealous, or worried, it means your brain is working just as it should, sending you important messages. Sometimes, these strong emotions can feel like they're taking over, especially when things get tricky with friends. But what if you could become a superhero, someone who knows when to pause, breathe, and choose a helpful response instead of reacting in a way that might hurt yourself or your friends?

Emotional regulation is a skill you can practice, like riding a bike or playing a game. It's not about being calm all the time or hiding your feelings, but about learning to handle them in ways that strengthen your friendships and help you feel proud of yourself. This chapter is packed with cool tools and fun challenges to help you become a friendship superstar! You'll learn how moving your body, eating well, and sleeping enough can help you become a master of your own emotions. Get ready to discover secret tricks, like superhero breathing and mood-boosting moves, that help you and your friends have the best adventures together.

DOI: 10.4324/9781003617570-2

Setting the scene (Self-Awareness, Empathy)

Imagine if you had a magic remote control for your feelings. When things get tricky at school, like when you feel left out at recess or have a disagreement with a friend, you could press pause, rewind, or even fast-forward to a happier moment! While we can't really press buttons, learning how to manage our feelings is the next best thing. When you understand your emotions and learn how to handle them, you can keep your friends close, even when things get tough.

Let's turn our feelings into friendship superpowers! By practising self-awareness (noticing how you feel), self-regulation (choosing how to act), and empathy (understanding others), you become the kind of friend everyone wants. Ready to power up your emotional intelligence and make every day at school a little more awesome?

Emotional intelligence starts in infancy and grows with us, shaped by genetics and experiences (Florida State College, 2016). Support from caregivers, life events and guidance all matter. Strong emotional intelligence means managing your own emotions and caring about others' feelings. Developing these skills takes time and practice (Brodie, 2025).

As children grow, they face situations needing emotional intelligence. Social awkwardness and misunderstandings are normal and can make resolving issues harder.

Emotional intelligence is self-awareness, self-regulation, empathy and social skills. These help us handle challenges with understanding and compassion. When friendships get tense, emotional intelligence helps manage emotions before they escalate. These skills are complex, even adults struggle with them, so lead with compassion and realistic expectations (Mattila et al., 2012).

Respectful conflict resolution is a major challenge in friendships (Collaborative for Academic, Social & Emotional Learning, 2024). Open, honest discussions help young people see conflict as normal and learn to handle it well (Office of Population Affairs, 2015).

Using emotional intelligence in hard moments builds trust and understanding, helping friendships grow through challenges rather than break down (Barrett, 2019).

Emotional regulation matters because our behaviour affects how safe others feel with us. People notice actions like yelling, nagging or being mean, even if we don't. Children want to be around gentle classmates who make them feel safe (Dehghani et al., 2022).

This chapter offers tools to build emotional intelligence. Approach this with compassion—these skills develop slowly, often into adulthood (Brodie, 2025; Hoet, 2023).

Spotting the skills in action (Observation and Reflection) (Self-Awareness, Empathy, Communication Skills)

Let's jump into a real-life story! Get ready to put on your detective hats and explore how feelings work in action

Micha's moment

Meet Micha—a boy who has more energy than a rocket! Before school, Micha zoomed around on his bike, climbed everything in sight, and played tag with friends. But once the bell rang, he had to sit still in class. Can you imagine having so much energy that it feels like you might burst? That's how Micha felt. He tried his best to sit quietly, but it was super hard, and it made it tricky to listen, learn, or keep his cool when things didn't go his way.

Sports day was coming, and Micha, the sports leader, was excited to present at assembly. After his usual energetic morning, the school lined up for the hall.

During the anthem, Micha enjoyed standing and singing, sneaking in a wriggle before sitting again.

Time crawled by as different speakers talked and talked. Micha wiggled in his seat, his excitement bubbling over into frustration. He wanted to be kind and patient, but it felt like he had ants in his pants! Waiting was the hardest thing ever for him.

Suddenly, Micha couldn't hold it in anymore. He blurted out, "blah blah blah, hurry up!" right in front of everyone! Some kids burst out laughing, others looked shocked. Micha was whisked off the stage, his face burning with embarrassment. A friend tried telling silly jokes to cheer him up, but Micha just wanted to disappear. Sometimes, big feelings come out in surprising ways!

After assembly, Micha felt exhausted and embarrassed. He ran laps to cool down, then bravely apologised to the other captain, who forgave him with a laugh.

Ask your students the following questions

Would you have forgiven Micah if you were the other captain? Why/why not?

Why do you think such a happy moment ended up in such a mess for Micah?

What feelings were hard for him to handle?

Were there any clues in the story that, no matter how happy Micah was at the assembly, it was very possible that something might go wrong?

What did Micah do right every day to help with his extra energy?

What did Micah do right on the day of the assembly?

If you were the teacher, what would you have done when Micah burst the words out at assembly?

What could happen differently to help someone like Micah?

Parent and educator reflection

How do you know a child is struggling with emotional regulation?

What are some of the less obvious reasons you've seen behind children struggling to regulate emotions?

What do you think about Micah and his excess energy?

Would you have handled the situation any differently as Micah and as the teacher?

How brain health helps with big feelings and how handling big feelings helps friendships (Self-Awareness, Emotional Regulation)

When friendship troubles pop up, it's easy to get stuck thinking about how much you're hurting, like there's a storm swirling in your brain! But here's a secret: if you give yourself a little time to cool off (like taking a brain break or a few deep breaths), you can come up with way better solutions than if you try to fix things while your feelings are still doing backflips.

A child's actions when frustrated don't reflect their true character. Brain health shapes mood, decisions and behaviour, but it's often overlooked (Dehghani et al., 2022). If a child struggles with emotions or friendships, consider brain health in support strategies. Genetics and personality affect self-regulation, but it's vital to model hope and focus on what's in our control. Habits, connections and environment can powerfully shape our growth (Hoet, 2023).

Good brain health helps us manage emotions and moods better (Dai & Ouyang, 2025)

Get your class talking: What happens when a small friendship problem suddenly feels HUGE because emotions are running wild? How can our words or actions in those moments sometimes make things even messier? Then, let's discover how taking care of your brain (with good food, sleep, and movement) can be like having a superpower for handling tough friendship moments! Use these questions to get everyone thinking and sharing their best ideas.

How would you know if your brain was healthy or unhealthy?
What helps build a healthier brain?
What do you think might make our brains unhealthier?
What brain fuel might help you with friendships?

Emphasise self-leadership: Improving brain health is always possible. Focus on what's in your control—movement, sleep, nutrition, creativity, and gratitude. Healthier brains make better decisions and handle emotions more effectively (Clark et al., 1999; Kok & Fredrickson, 2010).

Finding the right fuel for your brain

Nutrition, sleep, movement, and healthy habits look different for everyone. Empower young people to focus on what they can control for better brain health (Kok et al., 2013).

Would you?
Playfully ask your students:

Would you fill a Mercedes with sawdust instead of fuel?
Would you clean your PlayStation in a tub of water?
Would you feed
Would you leave your most treasured asset in the middle of a busy road?

Hand out poster-sized paper and divide the class into seven groups. Assign each group one of the situations that follow. Allow time to explore what a healthy and an unhealthy brain might do, then work together to draw a flowchart showing a healthy brain on one side and an unhealthy brain on the other, with both brains handling the situation they've been assigned.

How do you think a healthy brain vs an unhealthy brain handles the following situations?

1. Anger?
2. Someone being mean on purpose?
3. Coming last in a race?
4. Disagreeing with a friend?
5. Taking "no" for an answer?
6. Winding down to go to sleep?
7. Making a decision?

After the posters have been prepared for display, students can create short movie clips comparing healthy and unhealthy brains. Share with other classes and families to build on the whole-school culture of a strong friendship blueprint and the power of optimal brain health to help that happen. Students can teach their families what they have learnt (teaching someone a skill is one of the best ways to strengthen your own understanding of that skill).

Feelings are information. What are they trying to tell you? (Self-Awareness, Empathy)

Tough emotions like anger, anxiety and frustration show a strong, healthy brain (Brackett, 2019). We're meant to feel a full range of emotions; struggling to process them is a sign we need support.

Every emotion has a purpose, often linked to survival and social connection (Florida State College, 2016). Understanding and working with emotions is key to healthy friendships.

Let's have some fun! Split the class into pairs or small groups and give each group an emotion to become experts on. Your mission: Create a role play, write a funky rap, or design a colourful poster to teach the class all about your emotion. Get creative, costumes and silly voices encouraged!

Anger
Anger wants to protect you. It can be guided to solve the problem kindly, not hurtfully.

What it's telling you: Something feels unfair, or a boundary has been crossed.
What can help: Slow breaths, movement, music, pausing before saying or doing anything, and trying to talk only when you're calm.

Discussion and reflection
What does your body feel like when you're angry?
What can you do to calm down before you talk about it?
Can anger ever help us? When?

Anxiety (also known as worry)
What it's telling you: Your brain thinks there might be danger or something important to prepare for.
What to do: Start with a reality check. Is your worry real or a false alarm? Move your body by giving your stress and worry a "job". Stress and worry are created in our minds, so shifting our focus to our bodies

and releasing the energy of worry can help us calm down. Move by jumping up and down, doing a wall sit, running laps, playing sports, riding your bike, or doing some push-ups. Take a few slow, deep breaths, then take one small step forward with courage.

Discussion and reflection

What helps your body feel calm when you feel worried?

How can you tell if your worry is a true alarm or a false one?

Who helps you feel brave when you're scared?

Sadness

What it's telling you: You've lost something or someone important, or something didn't go the way you hoped.

What can help: Sadness can feel so horrible; you just want it to go away, but some feelings need time and need to be felt before you can move forward through them. It's okay to cry. Write or draw about it in a journal. Tell someone how you're feeling. Get busy with a hobby to give your brain a break and help you feel better.

Discussion and reflection

When have you felt sad, and when did someone help you feel better?

What kind of things can you do for yourself when you feel sad?

Why is it okay to cry?

Happiness

What it's telling you: Something feels good, safe, or meaningful right now.

What you can do: Notice and enjoy happiness, and share it. Write in a gratitude journal and appreciate your good moments.

Discussion and reflection

What makes you feel happy inside?

How can you help someone else feel happy, too?

What happens when we notice the small happy moments each day?

Excitement

What it's telling you: Something new or wonderful is about to happen!

What you can do: Use your energy wisely. Sometimes, excitement can build quickly, and we might find ourselves over-the-top or silly, which can frustrate the people around us. Take slow, deep breaths just like you would if you were angry or sad. Focus, and if your excitement has created extra energy, move.

Discussion and reflection

What exciting things have you looked forward to lately?

How does your body feel when you're excited?

What helps you stay calm enough to enjoy exciting moments?

Jealousy

What it's telling you: You see something someone else has, and you wish you had it too.

What might help: See jealousy as a clue to your own wishes. Use it to inspire you—not compare or criticise.

Discussion and reflection

When have you felt jealous of someone?

What can jealousy teach us about our own dreams?

How can we feel happy for others and still care for ourselves?

Disappointment

What it's telling you: Things didn't turn out how you hoped or planned, or you didn't get something you really wanted.

What to do: Feel disappointment, then look for lessons or try again. Plans rarely go perfectly, and that's normal.

Discussion and reflection

Can you remember a time you felt disappointed?

What helped you bounce back?

Why is it important to keep trying even when things don't go to plan?

Overwhelm
What it's telling you: You've got too much happening. Your brain and body need a break, fast.
What might help: Tell someone how you feel—sharing helps. Get enough sleep, move daily, drink water, make lists, and ask for help when needed.

Discussion and reflection
What helps you when you have too many things to think about?
How can you tell when you need a break?
Who can you ask for help when you feel overwhelmed?

Resentment
What it's telling you: You haven't felt treated fairly, or you are giving a lot to someone, and they are taking more than is fair.
What can help: Reflect on your needs—more help, rest, space, or boundaries. Resentment fades when needs are met and honesty is shared kindly.

Discussion and reflection
What happens when you keep saying "yes" but really mean "no"?
How can you ask for what you need in a kind way?
Why are clear boundaries important in friendships and families?

Feelings come from experiences that happen inside us and outside us. What experiences bring about your feelings? (Self-Awareness)

Feelings show a healthy brain, but handling them well is key to friendships and well-being. Every experience—thoughts, sights, sounds, events—can spark emotions.

When something bothers or excites us, emotions can escalate quickly.

There are also internal factors that can trigger us. Like thinking in an unhelpful way about our lives and other people. Doing this too often can create pathways for negativity in our minds, making it hard for us to see the beauty and wonder of life. Or, as we learned in the previous lesson, poor brain health can affect our mood and emotions, leading us to make bad decisions and experience irrational emotions that don't match our experiences (Sifferlin, 2015).

Brainstorm: Favourite, neutral, and least favourite experiences

Help students see that most feelings come from experiences, thoughts, or conversations. Pleasant experiences create good feelings; unpleasant ones create uncomfortable emotions. Some experiences are neutral.

Divide the whiteboard into three columns titled "favourite, neutral and least favourite." You can also use words like "positive, neutral and negative." Show face emojis that represent the three columns. Invite students to nominate their favourite, neutral and least favourite experiences and record their answers. For students who are less likely to put their hand up, ensure that you provide an opportunity to write or draw an answer and submit it to you.

Explain that the least favourite experiences are often called "triggers." Connect experiences to the emotions they cause.

You can share your own experiences that lead to your most uncomfortable emotions, like someone being dishonest, being interrupted constantly, or people being mean on purpose. You can even let your students interview you on the three columns for your own answers.

Let's play a feelings relay! After collecting everyone's examples, turn your classroom into a running game. When you hear a scenario, dash to the side of the room that matches how you feel—happy, sad or just "meh." If you're not sure, freeze in the middle! Get ready to laugh, think, and maybe even discover something new about your friends (and yourself).

When you join the shorter line for the canteen, the long line moves way faster ahead of you, and you're still standing there.

When you are doing a group assignment, and you're the only one doing the work.

When your teacher lets you out before the final bell.

When you have worked hard to build something, and it breaks.

When you win.

Christmas Day or other festive celebrations such as Wesak, Diwali, Chinese New Year or Ramadan.

When your eraser leaves a smudge instead of erasing.

When someone is out in a game, and you know for sure they're out, but they argue and refuse to go out.

Family holidays.

Swimming in the ocean.

Swimming in a pool.

Rainbows.

Thinking about a fight with a friend.

Rainy days.

When you are just getting to the best part in a video game, and you must stop to do your chores.

When grown-ups say, "because I said so."

When you find the perfect grassy hill to roll down with your friends, and there's a safety sign saying no to rolling down the hill.

Watching sport.

When you're in the middle of a great game and the bell goes.

When your favourite lesson is PE, and it's pouring with rain, you can't go outside, and need to do PE theory at your desk instead.

Role plays with a twist (Empathy, Perspective Taking, Communication Skills, Problem Solving)

Here's a twist on our role plays: Your job is to become an emotion detective! When someone in the role play is acting in a tricky or upset way, use your emotional intelligence superpowers to figure out what they might be thinking or feeling. Can you show empathy and help solve the problem kindly? If not, think of a courageous way to talk to them about how their actions are making others feel. Remember—real friends help each other grow!

You're playing cricket, you bowl the batter out, nice and clean, all three wickets are down. They tell you they weren't ready. They refuse to move off the pitch.

You've worked hard on a presentation and know you did an excellent job presenting it to your class. On your way back to your seat, you feel uncomfortable because your best friend stared out the window with a bored look on their face the whole time you were speaking.

Your friend comes over and tells you they've been invited to hang around with the very group that has excluded you and your friend all year. You don't have any other friends, and you're now on your own.

Another student calls out, laughing and making exaggerated yawn sounds during your solo rehearsal for the school concert.

You're waiting in line at the school tuck shop, and someone pushes in front of you and says, "Sorry, but I have a lunch meeting for school leaders and I'm late!" You're okay with that part, but you're not impressed that they didn't ask or check whether you were.

There's rain and clouds tumbling in the sky, and one of your friends has been complaining all day about how recess and lunch are ruined, and it's going to be the worst day ever. Hours before the rain turns up, he's brought it up what feels like a hundred times.

End the lesson with games that encourage students to notice their own and others' emotions as they win and lose.

Emotions and devices. A recipe for disaster? (Communication Skills, Emotional Regulation, Empathy, Conflict Resolution)

Children's use of devices often leads to miscommunication and overreactions (European Union, 2025; Ortutay, 2023). Written words can lack tone, and conflicts can continue after school. Sometimes devices are used to bully. Delaying device use gives brain more time to develop social skills.

Set clear boundaries for mobile device use before children get one, so they are prepared.

Invite your students to share their thoughts on the best and safest ways to use a device and to suggest ways to avoid social conflict (Figure 2.1).

Once you've shared these ideas with your class, they're ready to stretch their empathy muscles with role plays.

Assign one rule to each group and ask them to create role plays that address the associated questions.

ONLINE?

BE KIND, HAVE FUN, AND STAY SAFE.

Text to make plans or share smiles, **not to argue.**

Got a problem? Call or chat in person!

Stop and think before you post. Is it kind? Is it true? Is it needed? Only share if yes.

Give real compliments, share friendly jokes, and **make others smile.**

If you're upset, pause, put your device down, count to ten, or ask an adult for help.

Always ask before sharing photos or messages, **respect others' privacy.**

Group chats. **Include everyone** and keep it kind. If it turns mean, leave or speak up kindly.

Use kind emojis to share happy feelings. **Don't use emojis to tease** or be mean.

Take breaks from screens, move, play, and **talk with friends in person.**

Only share what's true, kind, and safe. Don't spread rumours or secrets.

Be kind online and offline, everyone has feelings, just like you.

If something feels wrong, tell a trusted adult. **You're never alone.**

1. ***Pause before you post***

   What could happen if you send a message when you're angry or upset?

   After you've answered, Role-Play typing an angry message, then deleting it and rewriting it in a kind manner. Talk about how that felt.

2. ***Use your words to lift people up***

   How can kind words change someone's day?

   Think of one kind message you could send to a friend right now or write in a card.

3. ***Don't reply in anger***

   You get a message that feels rude or unfair. What could you do instead of replying straight away?

   Share what helps you calm down before responding.

4. ***Respect people's privacy***

   Why is it important to ask before posting or sharing a photo?

   Role play: one person takes a photo, the other decides whether to give permission and why.

5. ***Be careful with group chats***

   A friend is being left out of the group chat. What could you say or do to include them?

   What does a respectful group chat look and sound like?

6. ***Use emojis wisely***

   Have you ever had someone misunderstand your message?

   Activity: Examine the same message with different emojis and discuss how each one alters the meaning.

7. ***Give your brain a break***

   How does too much screen time make you feel?

   Brainstorm fun "off-screen" things to do that make you feel good.

8. ***Think before forwarding or sharing***

   Someone sends you a funny video about a classmate. It's not kind. What could you do?

   What makes sharing "funny" things risky sometimes?

> **9. *Remember there's a real person behind every screen***
> How can we show empathy online?
> Practice turning a message that could sound harsh into one that feels gentle and caring.
> **10. *Ask for help if something feels wrong***
> Why is it brave to ask for help online, not weak?
> Create a list of trusted adults or friends you could go to if something online worries you.

Emotions and friendships: why handling feelings matters when friends disagree

During childhood, limited experience, underdeveloped emotional regulation skills and conflicting communication styles make disagreements between young people inevitable (Wang et al., 2025). Conflict and disagreements are great opportunities to develop perspective, practice self-regulation, enhance social awareness, and refine social and communication skills (Williams, 2025). These are tough skills to learn. Going through everyday misunderstandings, occasionally feeling left out, and experiencing changes in friendship dynamics provide perfect opportunities (with our support and guidance) to develop these skills. While these experiences are all painful, and we certainly don't want them to happen more than the joyful and mutually respectful interactions, early childhood is practice for the very real ups and downs of human relationships.

A peaceful society needs people who can adapt to different personalities and viewpoints (Iqbal et al., 2016). Respect, empathy, and self-regulation are crucial for navigating misunderstandings and differences in all relationships.

Missing out on a party hurts, but it teaches that not all relationships last (Barrett, 2019). With compassion, children can learn to accept change without taking it personally.

Stay compassionate—what seems minor to adults can feel huge to a child still learning about emotions and friendships (Hoet, 2023).

When emotions overwhelm us, we may make poor decisions (Brackett, 2019).

Explain these concepts to your students and help them understand further by sharing the following case study:

The day Mika was mean on purpose

Mika's best friend Jemima told her she couldn't come to her birthday party because she had brown skin and autism, and that she was sorry. Jemima said it was her parents' decision, not hers, and that she had a big argument with them. They said they would cancel her party if she kept arguing. Mika's mind focused on feeling left out and missing out on a party. Mika's feelings exploded out of her pores in her skin. She wanted to hurt Jemima back as much as she had hurt Mika. With her hot, angry head, she told Jemima's friend Nina that Jemima didn't want to invite her to the party either (which wasn't true). It didn't take long for Mika's teacher to notice there was arguing and tears in the playground. In the shame and embarrassment of that moment, Mika lied again and said Jemima had been bullying her all year, putting dirt in her school bag and being mean on purpose about her being brown and having autism. Jemima had never done any of this, and never would. The school bell rang, and their teacher said they would discuss it in the morning. Jemima could hardly breathe; she was crying so much that she could barely breathe. Nina didn't know what to believe, and Mika felt so sick in her tummy that she vomited in the car on the way home.

Mika begged her parents to stay home the next day, and they agreed. Jemima had cooled down by morning and was able to see things from Mika's perspective, understanding that feelings got in the way of kindness. She was ready to forgive, but Mika wasn't there.

Group discussion (Empathy, Perspective Taking, Communication Skills, Conflict Resolution)

Invite your students to share their opinion about how they would handle this situation if they were any of the characters. Write their ideas on the board.

Extend the discussion to consider other social situations in which people act out of character due to emotion and need to find the courage to make things better, or risk losing a precious friendship. Divide the class into pairs to role play new ideas and solutions.

Where emotions can take us and how to get stronger at handling them (Self-Awareness, Emotional Regulation, Conflict Resolution)

Big feelings often come with unhelpful thoughts. When emotions run high, it's hard to think ahead or consider consequences.

Time to get creative! Pick a scenario from the list and turn it into your own comic strip. Show what happens when big feelings arrive. Will your comic have a happy ending, a silly twist, or even a "whoops" moment where things don't go as planned? Draw the characters' faces and speech bubbles to show how everyone is feeling and what they could say or do next. When you're done, help make a class comic book so everyone can enjoy the stories and ideas!

1. ***The lunchtime dilemma***
   Scenario: You and your best friend always sit together at lunch. One day, they sit with someone else and don't save you a spot.
   Big Emotion: Rejection and sadness.
   Choices:

   a. Walk over and ask if you can join them.
   b. Sit alone and feel upset.
   c. Join another group at a nearby table.
   d. Ignore them for the rest of the day.

2. ***The group project trouble***
   Scenario: You're assigned to a group project, but one person is bossy and keeps telling everyone what to do. You feel frustrated and unheard.

Big Emotion: Anger and frustration.
Choices:

   a. Tell the teacher right away.
   b. Talk to the teammate and explain how you're feeling.
   c. Stay quiet and do what they say.
   d. Refuse to do the project.

3. The secret that spread

Scenario: You told a classmate something personal and asked them to keep it secret. Now others are whispering and laughing.

Big Emotion: Embarrassment and betrayal.
Choices:

   a. Confront your classmate and ask why they shared it.
   b. Tell the teacher what happened.
   c. Cry in the bathroom.
   d. Pretend it doesn't bother you.

4. The exclusion game

Scenario: You want to play a game during recess, but the other kids say, "You can't play with us today."

Big Emotion: Hurt and loneliness.
Choices:

   a. Ask why you can't play.
   b. Walk away and play alone.
   c. Find another group to play with.
   d. Shout, "You're mean!" and run off.

5. The broken promise

Scenario: A friend promised to partner with you for a class activity, but when the time comes, they choose someone else.

> *Big Emotion:* Disappointment and jealousy.
> *Choices:*
>
> a. Ask them why they changed their mind.
> b. Choose a new partner and let it go.
> c. Refuse to do the activity.
> d. Say something mean to your friend.

Emotional regulation tools to strengthen your vagus nerve (Emotional Regulation, Self-Awareness)

Lots of things, not just friendship problems, can make handling emotions tough. Sometimes it feels like you're a soda bottle that's been shaken up. But just like you can practice sports or music, you can practice calming down your big feelings. There's even a "superhighway" in your body (called the vagus nerve) that helps you calm down after excitement or stress. The more you practice, the easier it gets to feel cool, calm, and in control—even when things get wild!

Vagal tone refers to the functional state of this system and is often indexed by respiratory sinus arrhythmia (RSA), the natural variation in heart rate that occurs with breathing (Thayer et al., 2009).

Research by Stephen Porges (Polyvagal Theory) and others shows that high vagal tone is linked with greater emotional regulation, better social engagement, and faster physiological recovery after stress (Gillie & Thayer, 2014; Thayer et al., 2009).

Activities such as deep breathing, singing, humming, yoga, safe social connection, and even kind touch have been shown to improve vagal tone through increased parasympathetic activity (Gillie & Thayer, 2014; Kok & Fredrickson, 2010).

The superhighway in your body. An explanation for students to help them understand the vagus nerve

Imagine a secret road called the vagus nerve zooming from your brain to your heart, lungs, and tummy. It's like a special delivery service for calm feelings!

It acts as a walkie-talkie between your brain and body. When you feel calm and safe, your body relaxes and rests.

When you're scared or upset, your body prepares for danger. Afterwards, it helps you return to a calm state.

Vagal tone

"Vagal tone" is how strong and flexible the vagus nerve is (Thayer et al., 2009). Higher vagal tone helps you switch easily between excitement and calm—like a superhero relaxing after action. People with higher vagal tone feel calmer, handle big feelings better, get along with others and stay healthier (Gillie & Thayer, 2014; Kok & Fredrickson, 2010).

How to make your vagal tone strong

Slow breathing, exercise, laughter and connection help your vagus nerve signal safety, letting your body relax (Gillie & Thayer, 2014; Kok & Fredrickson, 2010).

Other ways to strengthen your emotional regulation skills

1. *Turtle Time (Emotional Regulation, Self-Awareness)*
   Try Turtle Time! When you feel upset, pretend you're a turtle. Pull into your shell by giving yourself a gentle hug, taking a few slow breaths, or finding a quiet spot. This gives your brain a chance to think and helps you handle your feelings like a pro.
2. *Grounding (Self-Awareness, Presence, Emotional Regulation)*
   Notice 5 things you can see, 4 things you can hear, three things you can touch, two things you can smell, and 1 thing you can taste.
3. *Pause. (Self-Awareness, Emotional Regulation)*
   When upset, it's hard to think. Take deep breaths, count to 10, pause before speaking, drink water, or splash cold water on your face before reacting.
4. *Use Kind Words, Not Blame. (Communication Skills, Emotional Regulation)*
   Mean words make things worse. Speak calmly and use "I" statements, such as "That hurt my feelings," rather than blaming.
5. *It's Okay to Take a Break. (Self-Awareness, Communication Skills)*
   Taking a break from a friend can help cool emotions. Let them know kindly: "I need a little break. Can we talk later?"

6. *Planning ahead and being prepared for big feelings.*
   Problems between friends often happen when emotions take over. Plan ahead to manage your feelings, and be gentle with yourself as you learn.

Journaling

Allow students time to write or draw in their notebooks about the tools they would like to try to manage their emotions in healthy, constructive ways. Ask them to create a drawing that explains the vagus nerve and to think of three situations in which they could use a strategy to regulate their emotions in the week ahead.

Key takeaways: Chapter 2: How emotional regulation helps friendships

- Emotional regulation is the ability to notice, understand, and manage our feelings, rather than letting emotions dictate our actions.
- Strong friendships depend on emotional intelligence, which includes self-awareness, self-regulation, empathy, and social skills.
- Managing emotions helps children stay connected to friends, even during disagreements or challenging times.
- Emotional intelligence is developed through experience, guidance, and practice, and continues to grow well into adulthood.
- Self-awareness helps us notice our triggers and reactions; self-regulation helps prevent impulsive or hurtful responses; empathy helps us understand others' perspectives.
- Brain health (supported by movement, sleep, water, and nutrition) is crucial for good emotional regulation and decision-making.
- All feelings, including anger, anxiety, sadness, jealousy, and disappointment, are normal and contain useful information. Learning to process and express these emotions safely is key.
- Experiences and thoughts (both positive and negative) trigger emotions. Recognising and preparing for emotional triggers helps students respond thoughtfully.
- Digital communication brings new challenges for emotional regulation. Children should pause before posting, use kind words, and seek help if something feels wrong online.

- Conflict, misunderstandings, and feeling left out are normal parts of friendship and provide valuable opportunities for growth in emotional intelligence.
- Practical tools like mindful breathing, journaling, the five-finger countdown, and taking a pause support self-regulation.
- Developing emotional regulation skills takes time, practice, and support from adults.

Call to action

Teach emotional literacy explicitly and weave it into everyday interactions. Encourage students to practice emotional regulation skills, such as noticing their feelings, choosing their responses thoughtfully and supporting others in doing the same. As adults, our leadership matters, and it's essential that we role model the skills we expect to see in them. Support family and school culture that values emotional intelligence and provide ample opportunities to develop it. Ask your students how they will use their emotional intelligence to build and strengthen their friendships this week. Notice when students use emotional intelligence and acknowledge its value.

References

Barrett, P. (2019). *Friends resilience*. Friendsresilience.org. https://friendsresilience.org/

Brackett, M. (2019). *Permission to feel*. Yale University Press. https://yalebooks.yale.edu/book/9780300234010/permission-feel

Brodie, K. (2025). *Emotional intelligence: The complete guide to EQ development*. Early Years TV. https://www.earlyyears.tv/emotional-intelligence-development-guide/

Clark, K. B., Naritoku, D. K., Smith, D. C., Browning, R. A., & Jensen, R. A. (1999). Enhanced recognition memory following vagus nerve stimulation in human subjects. *Nature Neuroscience, 2*(1), 94–98. https://doi.org/10.1038/4600

Collaborative for Academic, Social & Emotional Learning (2024). *Social emotional learning*. Sesd.org. https://www.sesd.org/about-usnew/departments/teaching-and-learning-department/student-services/social-emotional-learning

Dai, Y., & Ouyang, N. (2025). *Excessive screen time is associated with mental health problems and ADHD in US children and adolescents: Physical activity and sleep as parallel mediators*. ArXiv.org. https://arxiv.org/abs/2508.10062

Dehghani, A., Soltanian-Zadeh, H., & Hossein-Zadeh, G.-A. (2022). *Neural modulation enhancement using connectivity-based EEG neurofeedback with simultaneous fMRI for emotion regulation*. ArXiv.org. https://arxiv.org/abs/2204.01087

European Union. (2025). *The impact of cyberbullying on children's emotional well-being*. Better Internet for Kids. https://better-internet-for-kids.europa.eu/en/resource-directory/impact-cyberbullying-childrens-emotional-well-being

Florida State College. (2016). *Emotions and their development and regulation*. Child and Adolescent Psychology; Pressbooks. https://fscj.pressbooks.pub/childpsychology/chapter/emotions-and-their-development-and-regulation/

Gillie, B. L., & Thayer, J. F. (2014). Individual differences in resting heart rate variability and cognitive control in posttraumatic stress disorder. *Frontiers in Psychology, 5*, 758. https://doi.org/10.3389/fpsyg.2014.00758

Hoet, A. (2023). *Helping kids cope with strong emotions*. Kids Mental Health Foundation. https://www.kidsmentalhealthfoundation.org/mental-health-resources/behaviors-and-emotions/coping-with-strong-emotions

Iqbal, H., Neal, S., & Vincent, C. (2016). Children's friendships in super-diverse localities: Encounters with social and ethnic difference. *Childhood, 24*(1), 128–142. https://doi.org/10.1177/0907568216633741

Kok, B. E., Coffey, K. A., Cohn, M. A., Catalino, L. I., Vacharkulksemsuk, T., Algoe, S. B., Brantley, M., & Fredrickson, B. L. (2013). How positive emotions build physical health. *Psychological Science, 24*(7), 1123–1132. https://doi.org/10.1177/0956797612470827

Kok, B. E., & Fredrickson, B. L. (2010). Upward spirals of the heart: autonomic flexibility, as indexed by vagal tone, reciprocally and prospectively predicts positive emotions and social connectedness. *Biological psychology, 85*(3), 432–436. https://doi.org/10.1016/j.biopsycho.2010.09.005

Mattila, A. K., Pohjola, V., Suominen, A. L., Joukamaa, M., & Lahti, S. (2012). Difficulties in emotional regulation: Association with poorer oral health-related quality of life in the general population. *European Journal of Oral Sciences, 120*(3), 224–231. https://doi.org/10.1111/j.1600-0722.2012.00953.x

Office of Population Affairs. (2015). *Emotional Development | HHS Office of Population Affairs*. Opa.hhs.gov. https://opa.hhs.gov/adolescent-health/adolescent-development-explained/emotional-development

Ortutay, B. (2023, October 24). *States sue Meta claiming its social platforms are addictive and harm children's mental health*. AP News. https://apnews.com/article/metachildrenteensharmslawsuit-17858802d76143d358e38ee15150dc94

Rogelio, S., Karina, E., Xavier, S., Vanessa, N., & Elizabeth, K. (2025). Impacto de la Regulación Emocional en el Rendimiento Académico: Estrategias Psicoeducativas para la Educación Básica. *Revista Iberoamericana de La Educación, 9*(4), 55–83. https://doi.org/10.31876/rie.v9i4.323

Sifferlin, A. (2015, December 16). *Depression in preschool changes the brain, study shows*. TIME; Time. https://time.com/4150637/depression-preschool-brain/

Thayer, J. F., Hansen, A. L., Saus-Rose, E., & Johnsen, B. H. (2009). Heart rate variability, prefrontal neural function, and cognitive performance: The neurovisceral integration perspective on self-regulation, adaptation, and health. *Annals of Behavioral Medicine, 37*(2), 141–153. https://doi.org/10.1007/s12160-009-9101-z

Wang, L., Cui, R., Wan, N., & Hu, W. (2025). Reshaping the ability–strategy link in emotion regulation: The role of a structured picture-book intervention for preschoolers. *Behavioral Sciences, 15*(8), 1137–1137. https://doi.org/10.3390/bs15081137

Williams, N. (2025, September 16). *Teaching kids emotional intelligence to resolve conflicts: How Ser-Kallai supports emotional growth*. Ser-Kallai. https://serkallai.org/blog/teaching-kids-emotional-intelligence-to-resolve-conflicts-how-ser-kallai-supports-emotional-growth

Appendix: Make it stick! Impactful activities for supercharging emotional regulation and friendships

1. Friendship superhero badges

Invite students to create their own "Friendship Superpower" badge. They can design a symbol or character that represents their best emotional regulation skill—like "Captain Calm" or "Empathy Ninja." Display the badges on a classroom wall of fame!

2. Classroom feelings chart

Set up a colourful daily feelings chart with emojis. Each student can check in every morning and afternoon, helping everyone reflect on emotions and supporting classmates who might need encouragement.

3. Emotion charades

Act out different feelings (without words!) and have classmates guess the emotion. This sparks laughter and helps kids practice noticing body language and facial expressions.

4. Brain breaks party

Schedule quick "brain break" dance parties, stretches or mindfulness moments throughout the week. Connect each break to a strategy for emotional regulation, like deep belly breathing or movement.

5. The compliment chain

Start a chain reaction of kindness by having each student give a genuine compliment to a new classmate every day. Watch as positive feelings spread and friendships grow stronger!

6. The friendship journal

Encourage students to keep a special journal in which they draw or write about a time when they used emotional regulation to solve a friendship challenge. Sharing stories helps everyone learn from each other.

7. Family connection cards

Send home "Family Connection" cards with prompts for students to discuss emotional regulation skills with parents or caregivers. Examples: "Share a time you took a break before reacting," or "What's a family tradition that makes everyone feel better?"

8. Emotion detective mystery

Create a classroom mystery game where students solve "friendship puzzles" by using clues about feelings and choosing the best responses. Celebrate the best emotion detectives at the end!

9. *Whole-school kindness day*

Organise a day when students from all classes participate in activities that highlight emotional regulation and empathy, such as a gratitude wall, buddy games, and group challenges.

10. *Reflection celebration*

At the end of the chapter, hold a celebration where students share their favourite tool, story, or victory from practising emotional regulation. Give out "Friendship Growth" certificates to every student for their effort and courage!

These creative, hands-on ideas help students remember the chapter's lessons, build classroom spirit, and bring emotional regulation skills to life, in and out of school.

Friendship Superpowers Toolkit
Friendship Challenge: Your Mission!

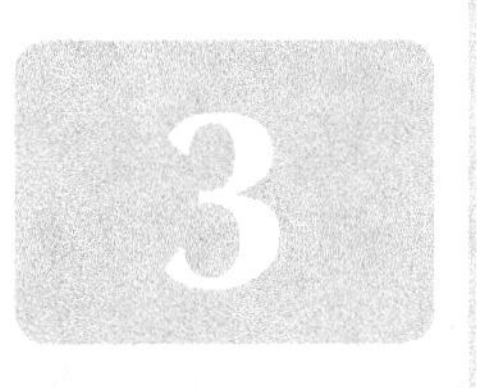

How overthinking friendships can burn out your friendship batteries

It's almost impossible for young people not to worry when friendships are challenging, but helping them to understand how worry can cloud judgement and use up their friendship batteries can help them develop a more proactive, solution focused response.

Friendship power quests

Let's turn learning into an adventure! Each lesson in this chapter becomes a quest, complete with challenges, games, and hands-on fun. The more students play, imagine and experiment, the more their friendship "superpowers" grow. Activities include:

Friendship detective: Solve playful mysteries about feelings and misunderstandings.
Kindness bingo: Complete a row by performing acts of kindness for classmates.
Energy charades: Act out what charges or drains a friendship battery.
Role-play rescues: Jump into silly or challenging friendship scenes and figure out ways to help everyone feel included.
Brain break battles: Quick, energetic games that help reset minds when overthinking strikes.

Each quest is designed to be short, exciting, and spark lots of laughter and reflection.

DOI: 10.4324/9781003617570-3

Before we dive in, let's explore why overthinking happens and how it drains our social energy (Lecce & Devine, 2021). Knowing this helps us get ready for the strategies and reflections coming up.

Many children, especially those who are sensitive, anxious, or neurodivergent, use up energy replaying conversations and worrying about mistakes (Smit et al., 2019). Caring is a strength, but overthinking can drain emotional energy and make friendships stressful. In this chapter, children learn to recognise signs of "friendship battery drain" and shift their focus to trust, curiosity, communication, and rest. Friendship should nourish, not exhaust.

This chapter helps children spot when they're overthinking, understand its impact, and use simple strategies to keep friendships healthy. They'll learn to distinguish between helpful reflection and unhelpful rumination, and practice ways to calm their minds, set boundaries, and build strong friendships.

Setting the scene

Friendships can be the best part about going to school, and they can also be the worst.

When friendships go well, they feel great; when things are off, they can cause anxiety and make some people reluctant to go to school. Upsets are normal, but young people, who are still learning to manage their emotions, can react with big feelings that affect their whole friendship group (Mittmann et al., 2022).

Intense emotions can lead to overwhelming thoughts, and as social beings wired for belonging, it's easy for friendship worries to take over (Lecce & Devine, 2021). This can make even small upsets feel huge, especially for children who are sensitive or anxious.

When social problems come up, children try to make sense of them. During tough times, automatic thoughts can lead to confusion and make things feel worse (Zainal & Newman, 2018). Young people often create explanations for their hurt, even when they aren't accurate. We all rely on family and community to thrive—real connections bring safety and belonging. Feeling connected at school through healthy relationships is essential for well-being (Mittmann et al., 2022).

As adults, our confidence and optimism in young people matter, along with our support in helping them find connection and belonging. Great friendships require many skills. Even when things go well, anxiety and overthinking can stop some children from enjoying friendships. This can lead to misunderstandings, conflict, and even compassion fatigue from peers (Smit et al., 2019).

Addressing overthinking helps students save emotional energy, enjoy happier friendships and focus on learning and growing (Mahoney et al., 2020). Managing overthinking builds resilience and supports strong friendships.

Spotting the skills in action (Observation and Reflection)

Let's jump into a real-life story! Get ready to put on your detective hats and explore how feelings work in action

Mia's emotional storm and overthinking nightmare

Mia arrived at the park with her Dad, bubbling with excitement to see her best friend Maneesha, just as they had promised each other the night before. They had Maneesha's favourite cupcakes and passed the time with eye spy, but every minute felt stretched and jittery. Five minutes in, dread tightened Mia's stomach. Her throat closed up; tears threatened; her mind raced with worry, a storm of anxious thoughts she couldn't calm. She felt panic thumping in her chest as each second passed. When Maneesha's Dad noticed her distress and asked if she was okay, the warmth in her own Dad's voice unlocked the floodgates. She sobbed into his arms. This storm wasn't new—each time, her thoughts spun darker, twisting every tiny uncertainty into something awful.

"What have I done?" "She's annoyed with me." "I knew something was wrong when she looked at me yesterday." "Ever since I started asking if we could play soccer some lunch times, she hasn't been the same. I should have stuck to her favourite, basketball." Why would Maneesha want to be friends with me when she is one of the most popular girls at school?" "What was I thinking coming here today? She was just being nice, saying she's come." "I can never keep new friends; I annoy everyone I ever meet." "Another reason to hate myself." "She's probably at that popular girls' party today." "Why did I ask her to meet anyway?" The tears rolled down almost as fast as the thoughts, while her Dad hugged her tight, without saying a word, and he didn't need to. A drizzle of calm trickled through, helping Mia slow her breathing.

Just as Mia calmed after crying, her dad put his hand on her heart and whispered, "Maneesha's here, sweetheart." Mia's heart filled with relief. She jumped up and hugged Maneesha as if they hadn't seen each other in years. Mia's emotions remained shaky, but she knew things were okay. Maneesha's Dad apologised for being late, and Mia's Dad laughed, saying, "It's only five minutes! Don't worry!" Five minutes? That's all!

Reflection for students

Did you think Maneesha would eventually turn up? Why/why not?

Why might five minutes feel like an eternity for Mia?

Can you think of a time when you or a friend imagined the worst, only for nothing to be wrong?

What could help stop these thoughts in their tracks?

Reflection for parents and educators

When have you noticed a child overthinking situations involving friendships?

Can you think of a time you were the "overthinker" either as a child or more recently as an adult?

How did it feel? What helped? What didn't help?

Have you noticed any similarities between the children who overthink and those who don't?

How do you know a student is an overthinker if they don't tell you directly?

Creating space between thoughts and emotions (Self-Awareness, Conflict Resolution, and Problem Solving)

Building on our observations, we'll now focus on practical strategies for managing overwhelming thoughts and emotions in friendships.

Our minds and bodies are deeply connected—unhappy events, especially ones that threaten our sense of belonging, often trigger unsettled, anxious thoughts and a strong biological response (Schneider et al., 2021). This "fight, flight or freeze" mode can make emotions feel overpowering and lead to chronic overthinking if we don't have strategies to manage it.

Giving time and space when emotions are high is the first step in helping the brain calm down and regain clarity. However, many young people react quickly and continue conflict through devices and group texts at home, which doesn't give their minds a break (Radesky et al., 2022). Unlike previous generations, today's children rarely get that pause to settle, which makes it harder to reset and repair relationships.

Group discussion: If the thoughts aren't helpful, move them on

In your own words, adapt the knowledge about how overthinking can happen easily, especially without a counter habit to help soothe emotions and interrupt the overthinking.

Invite your students to share their own ideas for creating space for emotions to settle and for helping them move through their bodies more constructively. Here are some ideas to teach your students and reflect on. (A shorter version is available in the poster set if you would like to incorporate this as a prompt.)

Move. The thinking part of the brain can't work properly when all the energy has gone into emotions. Getting out of your mind and into your body helps move upset energy, allowing the thinking part of your brain to switch back on.

Invite your students to answer the question, *"What are some ways you like to move? Could this help when you are having an emotional storm?"*

Give your stress "a job." Putting the extra emotional energy that emerges during stress into a "job" that helps take your mind off the situation can be a very helpful way to create time and space between an event and a response. Filling a drink bottle, watering a plant, shredding paperwork, practising soccer, writing friendly messages to family and friends, tidying up and decorating for a moment are all ways to use up the extra energy created by stress and frustration and put it towards something that feels great.

Ask your students, "What are more ways to give stress a "job?"

Tidying up and decorating were among the ideas on this list. Why do you think tidying up was included when most people don't even like tidying up?

Set a timer. Flip a sand timer or set a stopwatch for 5 minutes after something that upsets you happens, and try your best not to try to solve it, talk about it, say anything about it, or do anything about it in that time (unless it's an emergency, of course)! These precious five minutes give your brain a chance to slow down its survival response, tidy up thinking, and bring your wise and kind character back online. This means that whatever happens next will be kind to everyone involved, might lead to a great compromise or solution, and isn't an impulsive reaction.

> What could you use as a timer?
> Can you see how time could give you just the space you need for your brain to leave survival mode and re-enter connection mode?
> When would it not be a good idea or safe to wait 5 minutes before speaking or acting when you're emotional?

Think about something else for a while. It's very hard not to think about our problems, especially when we're still emotional. Usually, we think about our worries far more than is helpful. Trying to think about something else for a while—like your favourite places to visit, baby animals, your favourite movie, or person—can help your brain step out of survival mode and into relaxation mode. If this is very hard for you, try listening to music, podcasts, radio, or audiobooks to fill your mind with something else for a while. Overthinking something while you're upset will often make things worse and wire the wrong pathways in your beautiful brains!

What can you add to things to think about to help people stretch their imaginations and grow their toolbox of happy thoughts?

Try not to pick up a device—especially not to text the person you're upset with. Devices can feel soothing in the moment, but they release a burst of dopamine, and when you stop, your emotions can come crashing back (Doucleff, 2023). Instead, do something creative or active to help your mind reset.

Always remember that text messages are for planning social gatherings and other events, as well as for happy conversations; they are not for resolving conflicts.

> Has a device ever made feelings easier for you, and if so, what were you doing on it at the time?
> Has a device ever been the reason things got worse?

Sleep on it. Problems between people are the hardest kind of challenge, and that's why they can create the most amount of emotion and overthinking. Leaving a social problem for a few hours or a couple of days can make a significant difference in helping you move forward and upward. When you keep talking about a friendship worry after school through messages, especially when you involve another friend, and particularly when you're still emotional, you're dragging the feelings out longer than you need to. You can try to agree with your friend that if a real upset, like an argument, has come up, you will give each other some time and space. Agree on the time frame (e.g., one night, two days, or up to a week) before checking in with each other and moving forward or working on a solution.

Educators and parents, "leaving" a social complication behind for long enough that emotions settle, and logic enters is hard for anyone. For this generation, one of the biggest challenges is the sheer number of communication platforms available, without the need for face-to-face conversations (which require much more bravery). When a complex situation arises, children and teenagers can impulsively and reactively try to solve it through group or individual online chats. This approach often exacerbates the problems, especially when other children (and their parents) become involved. *

Students, why do you think experts recommend that text messages and group chats should only be used to organise and plan things, and conflict should only ever be resolved in person when emotions have settled?

> Has "sleeping on it," ever made things worse for you?
> Has "sleeping on it," ever made things better for you?

Moving unhelpful thoughts along the posters/pin-up board

Bring the ideas you have collaborated on through this discussion together and create a space to continue reinforcing them. As you know, children don't learn through one conversation and need many reminders (and a lot of modelling from adults) to develop a new skill.

An "I don't know that for sure" mindset to help with overthinking (Self-Awareness, Empathy and Perspective Taking, Communication Skills)

Overthinking is often an anxiety response—it pulls you out of the present, overestimates problems, and underestimates your ability to handle them (Zainal & Newman, 2018). For young people, whose brains are still growing, this can make social challenges feel even more overwhelming and threaten their sense of belonging.

An "I don't know that for sure" mindset is a powerful tool for responding to overthinking in a healthier, more balanced way. When valued friendships involve tough emotions, thoughts and feelings, they can quickly spiral out of control. Overthinking usually leads to different assumptions or misunderstandings. Shifting to an *"I don't know that for sure"* mindset can help students accept some ambiguity and recognise that not everything needs to be analysed or solved immediately. The "I don't know that for sure" approach also provides students with a self-talk script when they find themselves interpreting social situations based on their anxiety.

By embracing the uncertainty that's part of all relationships and letting go of trying to be aware of and in control of their friend's thoughts, moods and perspectives, students can reduce the pressure to interpret every action, word, or silence from a friend. This reduces anxiety and enables more natural and relaxed interactions. The "I don't know that for sure" approach fosters patience and openness, creating space for curiosity rather than judgement, encouraging them to trust the relationship rather than fixate on hypothetical problems.

Promoting healthier communication by thinking, "I don't know that for sure," helps students focus on the present, rather than ruminating over imagined scenarios. It invites students to seek clarity through honest dialogue, when necessary, rather than jumping to conclusions. In doing so, it prevents misunderstandings from growing into unnecessary conflicts.

Letting go of overthinking through an "I don't know that for sure" mindset helps friendships thrive in a more authentic, less pressured space, fostering deeper connection, trust, and emotional well-being.

> **Students**, remember Mia, who overthinks Maneesha coming late to the park? Think of a time you were worried about something that happened with your friend, and you started guessing what they were thinking and overthinking. Could the "I don't know that for sure," thinking (along with some quick emotional regulation tools) have helped you feel better?

"I don't know for sure," Role Plays

Once you've explained the "I don't know that for sure" mindset, and they've answered the questions, it's time to role-play and strengthen an "I don't know that for sure" mindset.

1. *The silent treatment*

   Scenario: You said something during lunch that made your friend go quiet. They haven't talked to you since. You start overthinking.

   Demonstrate how you can manage overthinking and worry, and provide a solution that is kind and considerate.

2. *The missed invite*

   Scenario: Your friend had a birthday party and didn't invite you. You're hurt, but also worried they're upset with you.

   Role-play how you slow your overthinking down and then express your feelings kindly with your friend and ask if something is wrong.

3. *The group project tension*

   Scenario: During a group project, you took charge, and now your friend seems annoyed.

   Role-play your thoughts, moving from catastrophic and self-critical to self-compassionate and calming, then explore how to apologise, include the other ideas, and move forward.

4. *The forgotten secret*

   Scenario: You accidentally told someone a secret your friend shared. Now they won't look at you. You are imagining they think you're the worst person in the world and that they are going to tell everyone to never be your friend.

Role-play how you get your thinking back on track, offer a sincere apology, and talk about how to rebuild trust.

5. *The swapped seat*

   Scenario: You sat next to someone else on the bus, and now your usual bus buddy seems upset. You notice they seem to be overthinking, and they look like they're about to cry.

   Role-play a gentle conversation to check in and explain.

6. *The changed plans*

   Scenario: You made plans with your friend, then cancelled to do something else. They're not talking to you now, and this has happened before. Your friend takes this kind of situation very personally, and you are also the kind of person who says yes straight away, then realises later you don't have the time to fit it in. It's nothing personal.

   Discuss how to show you still care and make it right.

7. *The misunderstood text*

   Scenario: You sent a message that your friend misread, and now they're ignoring you. This feels like the end of the world, and you're dreading talking to them about it because you think they won't listen or want to make things better with you.

   Practice shifting your overthinking and clarifying misunderstandings in a calm and kind manner.

8. *The laughing moment*

   Scenario: You laughed at something your friend did without meaning to be mean, but now they're hurt. You didn't realise this would upset them, and now you feel like you're a terrible person.

   Learn how to demonstrate empathy and clearly communicate your intentions.

9. *The one time team up*

   Scenario: You worked with someone else in P.E., and your friend feels left out. You don't like doing everything with the same person, and it's nothing personal, but your friend always chooses you above everyone else.

   Role-play ways to balance friendships and include while also keeping your boundaries.

What about the big feelings that show up when you're worried a friend is mad at you, and your mind imagines the worst?

Feelings can make it difficult to use strategies planned. While it's always good to have a plan and be prepared, it's important to give ourselves and our students permission to be human, because even the best-laid plans won't always unfold as we hoped. Strong emotions and challenging thoughts during a social difficulty are a sign of a healthy brain and a genuine concern for something that matters to them. Remind students they don't have to believe everything they think (because it's usually not true when combined with intense upsets), and that stressed bodies tune into stressed thoughts, which together make things even more overwhelming.

After explaining this to your students, share the blueprint poster on friendships and emotions to help with emotional regulation as a foundation for brainstorming and gathering healthier, more constructive thinking and stronger emotional regulation tools (Figure 3.1).

Understanding each other (instead of overthinking differences and catastrophising) (Empathy and Perspective Taking, Communication Skills)

Schools and classrooms are ideal places for students to practice understanding, accepting, and navigating different personalities (Koç et al., 2024). Building empathy and compassion takes time, patience, repetition and strong role modelling, not just one lesson.

Exposure to diverse communities early in life builds a strong social knowledge base (Koç et al., 2024). Normalising the "grey areas" of perspectives and values is crucial for social-emotional well-being (Li & Shum, 2025). When we don't have this knowledge, it's easy to become frustrated and resentful when faced with differences. Responding with kindness and respect, even when values clash, takes courage and humility. Overthinking other people's character and values uses up precious energy that's better invested in joy, connection, and well-being.

BIG FEELINGS?

TAKE A BREATH, STAY COOL AND KEEP YOUR FRIENDS.

1 **Breathe deeply.**
Stop and take 3 deep breaths before you talk, this helps you choose kind words.

2 **Check the facts.**
Our brains sometimes get mixed up. Ask yourself: "Did they definitely say they're mad?" or "Could there be another reason?"

3 **Use "I feel…" to share your own feelings.**
Don't guess what others feel, just say how you feel. "I feel sad because I care about us."

4 **Ask questions. Don't guess.**
Maybe they're just tired, not mad. Say: "Are we okay?"

5 **If you hurt someone, say sorry.**
A real apology means you know what you did, you feel sorry, and you want to make it better. "I'm sorry for what I said. I didn't want to hurt you."

6 **Give your friend space if they need it.**
If your friend needs a break, let them have it. Tell them you're ready to talk when they are.

7 **Ask a trusted adult for help anytime you feel stuck.**
Not sure what to do? Talk to a teacher or grown-up. You don't have to figure it out alone.

8 **Write your feelings or a note if talking is hard.**
If talking feels hard, write a note or your feelings first. Read it over and keep it kind.

9 **Be kind to yourself, everyone makes mistakes.**
Forgive yourself, and remember: being a good friend takes practice.

10 **One mistake doesn't ruin a friendship.**
Strong friendships get through tough times. A kind chat helps clear things up.

After summarising with your students, hand out paper and markers and offer the following reflection opportunity:

Think of a time you strongly cared about something, and someone you cared about disagreed.

Write and draw about what happened, how you felt, what helped, and what didn't help with moving forward.

A "rainbow mindset" framework for getting along, instead of overthinking differences

Getting along with a wide range of personalities and values is hard—even for adults! For students, starting a new class with different peers or teachers can feel daunting, especially if they face personality clashes or feel like they only have one friend. Educators carefully consider class placements, but the process is complex. For neurodivergent children, extra support or changes may be needed since our systems still mostly cater to neurotypical brains.

Often, it's safe and important to normalise the disappointment and uncertainty of new peers and teachers. Psychologists refer to this process as the "prosocial differentiation tolerance." Put simply, this is the ability to maintain empathy, cooperation and mutual respect despite individual differences.

Drawing on Social and Emotional Learning (SEL) principles (CASEL, 2020), Theory of Mind development (Premack & Woodruff, 1978; Wellman, 2014) and empathy neuroscience (Decety & Jackson, 2004), the Rainbow Framework in this lesson integrates key processes that support prosocial behaviour across personality and value differences (Mahoney et al., 2020) (Figure 3.2).

Building a rainbow mindset to get along rather than overthinking differences

Introduce the concept of the mind as a colourful rainbow. Thoughts, feelings, and your purpose form the colours, and no two mindsets' rainbows are the same. When people combine their own and other people's colours respectfully and kindly, making and keeping friends becomes easier, and deep learning about each other becomes possible.

Hand out notebooks or paper, and invite students to draw a nice, big rainbow with space to write in each colour. The colours are red, orange, yellow,

FRIENDSHIP RAINBOW

SHINE BRIGHT, EVERYONE BELONGS.

RED RESPECT

Everyone is unique and belongs.

We're all different, and that's good!
Notice and respect differences.
"I like my way, they like theirs."

ORANGE CURIOUS?

Ask questions and learn.

Ask, don't assume, don't judge.
Everyone thinks differently.
"I wonder why," not get mad.

YELLOW KINDNESS

Use kind words to help everyone feel happy and safe.

Use kind words, even if you disagree.
"I use kind words, even if I disagree."

GREEN FLEXIBILITY

Try new ways, and remember, there's more than one right answer.

Be willing to change and try again.
There's more than one right way.
"We can both be right."

BLUE CALM

Take a deep breath and be a friendly problem-solver.

Breathe before you speak.
"I breathe deep to keep my words kind."
Stay calm to solve problems
and keep friends.

When we use all these colours, respect, curiosity, kindness, flexibility, and calm, our friendship rainbow shines, even if we're different.

green, and blue. Explain how each colour will have a mindset tool to help make getting along with each other easier.

One by one, explain each colour, inviting them to draw or write their understanding of it. Make sure you are role-modelling as you teach by filling in your rainbow or having a pre-prepared one ready to show them. If you're feeling creative, use a big wall in your room to replicate this rainbow and fill it with the ideas you and your class come up with.

Rainbow check in

Display the poster in the classroom and yard, model the values, and help students remember the perspective next time they overthink personality, character, and value differences from peers. Disagreement and personal differences can be better resolved through questions like:

"Which colour do I need right now?"
"What colour could help our friendship?"
"Can I mix my colour with theirs to make something new?"

Here's how this might look: "I'm red because I want my way. They're blue because they want to be calm. Perhaps we can mix and create a purple shade? We can take turns."

Rainbow framework role plays

Using the rainbow framework, encourage your students to create role-plays to explore mutual respect, even amid our differences.

The lunchbox surprise

Scenario: Sam brings sushi to school. Mia says, "Ew, that's gross!" Sam feels embarrassed.
How can Mia learn that different families enjoy different foods, and that's okay?

The gaming disagreement

Scenario: Alex thinks violent video games are fun. Charlie says their parents don't let them play those because they value kindness.

Practice listening without judging or trying to convince the other person they're "wrong."

Celebrations

Scenario: Bella celebrates Christmas, while Noor celebrates Eid. Bella says, "Why don't you do Christmas? That's weird."

Find ways to respect different cultural and religious celebrations and find common ground.

The point of learning

Scenario: Liam thinks getting good grades is the most important thing. Jaya thinks that enjoying learning is more important than getting good marks.

Explore how different values lead to different behaviours and find a way to discuss them respectfully.

After-school fun

Scenario: One student prefers quiet hobbies, such as reading. Another loves noisy sports. They start teasing each other about it.

Create a role play where differences in personality and interests are celebrated, rather than mocking them.

Fashion opinions

Scenario: Taylor wears clothes from second-hand shops. Blake says, "That's weird. Don't you want something new that no one else has worn?"

Role-play how different values (like sustainability or trends) guide choices and why it's okay to follow either.

Pet talk

Scenario: One student believes animals shouldn't be kept as pets and follows a vegan lifestyle. Another thinks pets are part of the family and eats meat.

Role play how to listen to each other's beliefs and values kindly, without trying to "win" the argument.

Screen time debate

Scenario: Ava isn't allowed to use social media, but Jess is, and thinks Ava's
parents are too strict. Jess tells Ava it's going to be hard to stay friends if
she doesn't get social media, as she is missing out on all the conversations
that happen there.
Role play understanding families have different values and rules that don't
make one better than the other, and find a way to stay in touch without
using social media.

What makes a family?

Scenario: Kai mentions he has two mums. A classmate says, "That's not normal."
Role-play learning to respect diverse family structures and what makes a
family strong (which is love and care, not just structure).

The group project

Scenario: In a group project, one student wants everything to be perfect and
follows the rules strictly. Another prefers greater flexibility and creativity.
Role play valuing different ways of doing things and working together by
appreciating both structure and freedom.

What if my overthinking has some truth in it? Understanding non-verbal cues (Self-Awareness, Communication Skills, Empathy, and Perspective Taking)

Some friendship challenges stem from misunderstandings and difficulties
interpreting nonverbal communication. Sometimes a child's behaviour
needs guidance because they unintentionally upset others or miss social
cues that are reasonable and fair for another person's boundaries. Children
who struggle to pick up on these cues can find themselves upset about struggling friendships and unable to see that they might be able to do something about it if they apply self-awareness and social awareness. Sometimes
non-verbal cues are interpreted as bullying when, in fact, a child is doing
their best, despite the other child not noticing, to set a boundary.

Share the following poster and create Role-Plays to help them develop
stronger social awareness (Figure 3.3).

NEED SPACE OR WANT TO TALK?

LOOK FOR CLUES FROM YOUR FRIENDS.

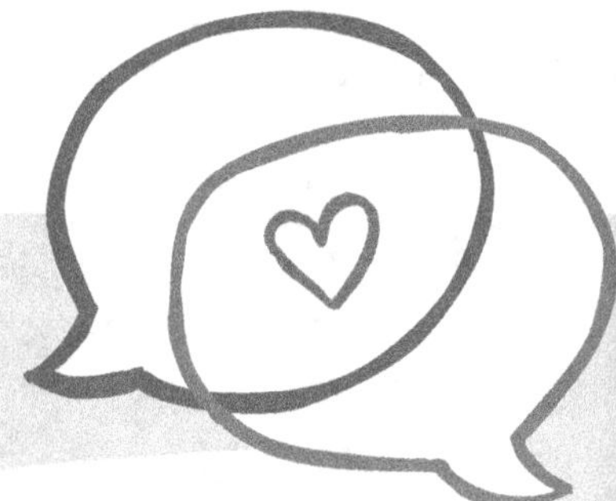

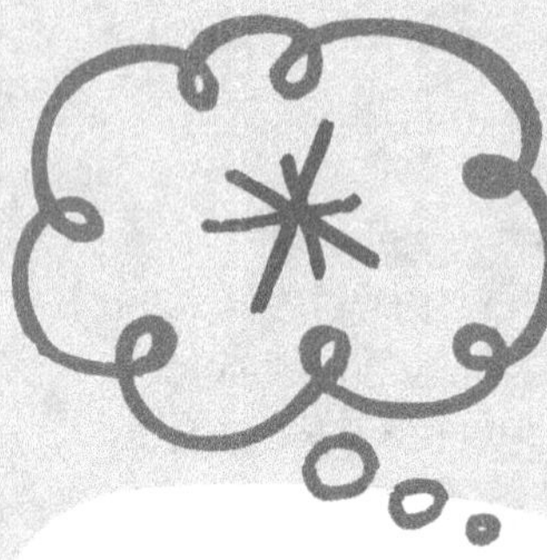

NOT SURE WHAT YOUR FRIEND NEEDS?
HERE'S HOW TO FIND OUT.

- They avoid eye contact or look away.
- They give short answers like, "I'm fine."
- They seem upset but won't explain why.
- They walk away or don't answer.
- They say, "Can we talk later?" or "I need a break."

WHAT YOU CAN DO:

- Say something kind like, "I'm here when you're ready." Give them time and space.
- Give them space and check in later.

SIGNS YOUR FRIEND WANTS TO TALK:

- They look at you, as if waiting for you to speak.
- They're quiet, but stay close.
- They seem sad or confused and aren't talking to anyone.
- They answer if you gently ask, "Are you okay?"
- They say, "That hurt my feelings," or "Why did you do that?"

WHAT YOU CAN DO:

- Be brave and kind. Say, "I feel like something's wrong. Can we talk?" Listen carefully, even if it's hard.
- If you're not sure, just ask kindly:
- "Want to talk now or need space?"
- This shows you care and respect their choice. Good friends help each other feel safe.

Students, can you think of any other signs someone might need space or wants to talk? Do you have any other ideas to help?

Protecting your friendship battery (Self-Awareness, Conflict Resolution and Problem Solving, Empathy, and Perspective Taking)

Each day, we have a limited amount of energy for learning, socialising, movement, and feelings. Kind and respectful friendships recharge us, while tricky social situations can drain our friendship battery quickly. It's important for students to learn how to be around people they don't always get along with, since everyone is learning and growing at their own pace. Adaptability and flexibility are key, and students will continue to build these skills throughout "The Friendship Blueprint."

Friendship battery game: Charge up or drain?

Create two signs, "energiser" and "drainer" and mark two sides of the room to represent each.
Show the "Charging up friendships" poster.

Invite students to create one simple scenario each of an everyday social situation between two or more people that is potentially draining but can be neutral or energising if handled with adaptability, kindness and flexibility. If you prefer, you can create situations based on what you have observed amongst peers, for example, two friends want to play, but they don't like the game the other person has chosen. Students seek a flexible solution that is energising, and facilitators help highlight adaptability over winning.

Set the scene

"We all have a *friendship battery*. Some conversations and interactions fill us up. Some drain us. Flexibility and kindness help everyone's battery stay healthy."

Students stand in a circle.
The teacher reads or shows a scenario card.
Students move to either the **ENERGISER** or **DRAINER** side of the room.

HOW FULL IS YOUR FRIENDSHIP BATTERY?

CHECK YOUR FRIENDSHIP ENERGY.

FULL + GLOWING

Friendship supercharged.

Warmth, kindness, listening, sharing, and smiles fill your battery.

CHARGING

Making things better: repairing your friendship.

Make space, say sorry, try again, and show you want to do better.

LOW

Running low: be kind to yourself and others to recharge.

Sulking, not sharing, complaining, arguing, or eye rolling drains energy.

FLAT

Out of energy: time to rest and recharge.

Arguing, pushing, shouting, blaming, or avoiding accountability drains your battery.

BE AN ENERGISER

Fill up your friendship battery by...

- ✓ Being kind.
- ✓ Using friendly words.
- ✓ Welcoming new ideas.
- ✓ Showing flexibility.
- ✓ Checking in: "Are you ok?"

DON'T BE A DRAINER

Keep your friendship battery full by avoiding...

- ✗ Taking over.
- ✗ Not listening.
- ✗ Only wanting your way.
- ✗ Leaving others out.
- ✗ Using a bossy tone.

Everyone gets tired sometimes. What matters is noticing, fixing, and recharging. We might not always get along, but we can always listen, learn, and try again.

Students share *why* and if it was a drainer, ask, "How could we change this, so it *fills* the friendship battery?" Use the battery visual as a reminder of where on the battery the situation and resolution might fit to keep the metaphor alive and visible.

Before sharing the poster that follows, highlight how healthy friendships need energy, not unnecessary mental checking, worrying, or self-doubt (Smit et al., 2019) (Figure 3.4).

Making our own friendship batteries

Hand out notebooks or paper so students can draw their own friendship battery. Remind them that investing energy in healthy friendships brings joy and energy to each day. Putting lots of energy into friendships that aren't a good match can feel draining. Overthinking and expecting everyone to think and feel the same way can lead to conflict and distance.

Key takeaways: Chapter 3: How overthinking friendships can burn out your friendship batteries

- Overthinking drains emotional energy and makes friendships feel exhausting instead of nourishing.
- Recognising and managing overthinking helps students conserve energy, reduce anxiety, and strengthen friendships.
- When students distinguish between helpful reflection and unhelpful rumination, using strategies such as movement, creative activities, and taking breaks, calm is much easier to restore.
- Emotional storms are normal, especially in young people, but practical strategies (like giving stress a job, using timers, and "sleeping on it") can help manage reactions.
- Adopting an "I don't know for sure" mindset helps challenge anxious thoughts and encourages clearer, kinder communication.
- The Rainbow Mindset Framework (Respect, Curiosity, Kindness, Flexibility, Calm) supports getting along with diverse personalities and values.
- Students practice empathy, perspective-taking, and social boundaries, learning to interpret non-verbal cues and respond to friends' needs for space or support.

- Adaptability and flexibility are emphasised as essential skills for maintaining healthy, balanced friendships and protecting one's "friendship battery."
- The chapter aligns with Australian Curriculum requirements by promoting self-awareness, emotional regulation, resilience, positive relationships, and social-emotional well-being.

References

Collaborative for Academic, Social, and Emotional Learning. (2020). *What is the CASEL framework?* https://casel.org/what-is-the-casel-framework/

Decety, J., & Jackson, P. L. (2004). The functional architecture of human empathy. *Behavioral and Cognitive Neuroscience Reviews*, *3*(2), 71–100. https://doi.org/10.1177/1534582304267187

Doucleff, M. (2023, June 12). *"Anti-dopamine parenting" can curb a kid's craving for screens or sweets*. NPR. https://www.npr.org/sections/health-shots/2023/06/12/1180867083/tips-to-outsmart-dopamine-unhook-kids-from-screens-sweets

Koç, S., Altınay, F., Koç, A., Altınay, Z., & Dagli, G. (2024). Cooperation of emotional intelligence and social activities in education: Effects on school culture and value acquisition. *Sustainability*, *16*(14), 6022–6022. https://doi.org/10.3390/su16146022

Lecce, S., & Devine, R. T. (2021). Social Interaction in early and middle childhood: The role of theory of mind. *Academic.oup.com*. https://doi.org/10.1093/oso/9780198843290.003.0003

Li, J., & Shum, K. K. (2025). Exploring the relationships between theory of mind, social skills, and friendship quality in adolescents and adults with and without autism spectrum disorder through structural equation modeling. *Journal of Autism and Developmental Disorders*. https://doi.org/10.1007/s10803-025-07039-9

Mahoney, J. L., Weissberg, R. P., Greenberg, M. T., Dusenbury, L., Jagers, R. J., Niemi, K., Schlinger, M., Schlund, J., Shriver, T. P., VanAusdal, K., & Yoder, N. (2020, October 8). Systemic social and emotional learning: promoting educational success for all preschool to high school students. *American Psychologist*. Advance online publication. http://dx.doi.org/10.1037/amp0000701

Mittmann, G., Barnard, A., Krammer, I., Martins, D., & Dias, J. (2022). LINA - A social augmented reality game around mental health, supporting real-world connection and sense of belonging for early adolescents. *Proceedings of the ACM on Human-Computer Interaction*, *6*(CHI PLAY), 1–21. https://doi.org/10.1145/3549505

Premack, D., & Woodruff, G. (1978). Does the chimpanzee have a theory of mind? *Behavioral and Brain Sciences*, *1*(4), 515–526. https://doi.org/10.1017/S0140525X00076512

Radesky, J. S., Kaciroti, N., Weeks, H. M., Schaller, A., & Miller, A. L. (2022). Longitudinal associations between use of mobile devices for calming and emotional reactivity and executive functioning in children aged 3 to 5 years. *JAMA Pediatrics*, *177*(1). https://doi.org/10.1001/jamapediatrics.2022.4793

Schneider, N., Greenstreet, E., & Deoni, S. C. L. (2021). Connecting inside out: Development of the social brain in infants and toddlers with a focus on myelination as a marker of brain maturation. *Child Development, 93*(2). https://doi.org/10.1111/cdev.13649

Smit, L., Knoors, H., Hermans, D., Verhoeven, L., & Vissers, C. (2019). The interplay between theory of mind and social emotional functioning in adolescents with communication and language problems. *Frontiers in Psychology, 10*. https://doi.org/10.3389/fpsyg.2019.01488

Wellman, H. M. (2014). *Making minds: How theory of mind develops*. Oxford University Press.

Zainal, N. H., & Newman, M. G. (2018). Worry amplifies theory-of-mind reasoning for negatively valenced social stimuli in generalized anxiety disorder. *Journal of Affective Disorders, 227*, 824–833. https://doi.org/10.1016/j.jad.2017.11.084

Appendix: Friendship power-ups toolkit

This appendix is a treasure chest for educators, packed with practical tools, playful printables, and memorable activities to make the lessons of Chapter 3 stick. Revisit it any time you need a quick boost for your classroom community!

1. Friendship battery tracker (printable): Let students colour in their battery level each morning and after key social moments. Use it for daily check-ins and class discussions on what helps charge or drain the group's energy.

2. Overthinking busters card deck: A printable set of cards with prompts like: "Name 3 things you like about yourself," "Tell a silly story about a time you worried for no reason," or "Invent a superhero who defeats overthinking!" Draw one whenever students get stuck in worry loops.

3. Friendship scenario dice: Create giant dice with friendship scenarios or emotions on each side. Roll and act out what could happen, focusing on flexible and positive responses.

4. Rainbow mindset colouring sheets: Let students illustrate the five friendship rainbow colours and write or draw examples of respect, curiosity, kindness, flexibility, and calm.

5. Energiser and drainer sorting game: Mix up cards with common school situations. Students race to sort them into "Energiser" or "Drainer" piles, then brainstorm ways to turn drainers into energisers.

6. Ready-to-use class posters: Printable reminders for "I Don't Know That For Sure" thinking, battery-charging behaviours, and the Rainbow Friendship Framework.
7. Educator reflection prompts: Quick questions and templates for teachers to jot down observations, student growth, or tricky moments—helpful for planning, reporting and supporting individual needs.

Return to this appendix whenever you want to refresh your classroom, reignite student engagement, or deepen the impact of your friendship lessons!

The red, green, and amber friendship lights

Learning quest: The friendship traffic light challenge! (Self-Awareness, Empathy, and Perspective Taking)

Get ready for a friendship adventure! Did you know friendships have their own secret signals, just like traffic lights? Learning to spot these signals can help you choose friends who make you feel happy, safe, and ready for fun!

Children are told to "be nice" or "be friends with everyone," but are seldom taught how to spot healthy, confusing, or unsafe friendships (Champlin, 2020; Rose & Rudolph, 2006). The red, green, and amber lights model offers clear language: green means safe and respectful; amber signals mixed or confusing feelings; red means uncomfortable or unsafe (Eisenberg et al., 2002). This chapter guides children to notice and trust their feelings, especially when friendships get complicated.

In this exciting chapter, you'll become a Friendship Detective! You'll learn how to spot green-light friends (super safe and kind), amber-light friends (sometimes tricky or confusing), and red-light friends (not safe or fair). Through fun stories and games, you'll practice picking the best friends, setting kind boundaries, and even being the kind of friend everyone wants to have. By the end, you'll have superhero friendship skills to help everyone feel included, confident, and happy!

DOI: 10.4324/9781003617570-4

Setting the scene: The great friendship adventure! (Self-Awareness, Communication Skills)

Relationships are shaped by our need for connection, belonging, and purpose (Eisenberg et al., 2002).

Our experiences and temperament shape how we see ourselves and others (Champlin, 2020).

To thrive, we need self-understanding, empathy, and community. The traffic light framework gives young people a practical tool for assessing friendships (Yong, 2008).

Green light behaviours show mutual respect, trust, and kindness. These friendships feel safe, supportive, and open—fostering emotional resilience (Eisenberg et al., 2002).

Red light behaviours signal harm: exclusion, bullying, controlling behaviour, lack of trust, or pressure to fit in. Friendships causing distress or anxiety are unhealthy (Jones & Rutland, 2019; Rubin et al., 2006).

Amber lights highlight grey areas—misunderstandings, social clumsiness, or one-time mistakes. They remind us to stay curious and open-minded as we navigate friendships (Champlin, 2020).

Promoting green lights and addressing red ones helps children build strong, positive friendships (Eisenberg et al., 2002).

This chapter clarifies which relationships are genuine and worth pursuing, highlighting the difference between trustworthy and complex friendships. It encourages students to stay open and curious as they navigate social relationships (Jones & Rutland, 2019).

If unsure what's age-appropriate, use the framework below. Everyone develops at their own pace, influenced by neurodivergence and environment (Champlin, 2020).

Early childhood (Ages 2–5)

Green light behaviours

Kindness and empathy: Around age 2, children begin to show empathy, though it is usually self-focused (Champlin, 2020).

Turn-taking and sharing: Sharing and turn-taking emerge around age 3–4 but may not be consistent until 7–8 (Yong, 2008).

Emotional regulation: Young children are still learning to manage emotions; by age 5, they have better control (Champlin, 2020).

Red/amber light behaviours

Aggression: Hitting or pushing is common at ages 2–3 due to developing impulse control; persisting after age 4 may require attention (Champlin, 2020).

Difficulty with sharing: Occasional sharing struggles are normal, but ongoing refusal may signal emotional or attachment challenges (Champlin, 2020).

Middle childhood (Ages 6–9)

Green light behaviour

Empathy and prosocial behaviour: By age 7, empathy grows more sophisticated, with children engaging in cooperative play and valuing fairness (Yong, 2008).

Positive communication: Children this age are developing better verbal communication skills and using words to resolve conflicts.

Respect for boundaries: Children around 7–8 years old can begin to respect personal boundaries and understand concepts such as consent and privacy.

Red light behaviour

Exclusion or bullying: Frequent exclusion or meanness at age 7–8 may signal bullying (Jones & Rutland, 2019).

Social isolation: Ongoing isolation or rejection at this age could indicate relationship or developmental challenges (Jones & Rutland, 2019).

Pre-adolescence (Ages 10–12)

Green light behaviour

Deeper friendships: By age 11, friendships become more emotionally supportive and loyal (Eisenberg et al., 2002).

Conflict resolution: Children can negotiate and compromise more effectively at this age (Eisenberg et al., 2002).

Mutual respect: Children become more sensitive to fairness and equity in friendships (Yong, 2008).

Red light behaviour

Cliques and exclusion: Habitual exclusion or gossip at age 10–11 may signal unhealthy dynamics (Jones & Rutland, 2019).

Dishonesty or manipulation: Pre-adolescents may test boundaries, leading to dishonesty or manipulation if values aren't developed (Eisenberg et al., 2002).

Adolescence (ages 11+ and what follows is looking more closely at 13 and up)

Green light behaviour

Emotional intimacy: Adolescents form deeper friendships, characterised by trust and emotional support (Champlin, 2020).

Identity exploration: Friendships help explore identity and values at this stage (Champlin, 2020).

Healthy boundaries and communication: Teens develop better skills for expressing needs and setting boundaries (Yong, 2008).

Red light behaviour

Toxic friendships: Adolescents may be vulnerable to toxic dynamics like manipulation, jealousy, or peer pressure (Jones & Rutland, 2019).

Constant conflict or aggression: Frequent conflict may signal issues with emotional regulation or peer pressure (Eisenberg et al., 2002).

At any age, red flags require reflection and, if needed, support. Childhood is the most powerful time to establish healthy social foundations (Champlin, 2020).

Spotting the skill in action (Observation and Reflection) (Empathy and Perspective Taking, Self-Awareness)

Let's jump into a story! Imagine YOU are the hero in this friendship quest. As you read, think about which friends are green, amber, or red lights. Ready? Let's go!

Albert's first day

When Albert's parents told him they were moving to another state, he felt like his whole world had cracked open. He loved his home, his school, and the friends he'd known since he was 5. On his last day, his classmates made a big arch with their hands and cheered as he walked out the gate. Albert cried so hard he thought his heart might break.

"I'll never find friends like them again," he whispered.

When Albert arrived at his new school, his stomach fluttered like a hundred butterflies. Everything felt different. The uniforms, the playground, even the smell of the classrooms. Albert decided to be brave and start this new chapter with an open heart.

On his first day, Albert met **Billy**, **Georgie**, and **Max**.

Billy smiled the moment Albert sat down. "Want me to show you around?" he said.

He pointed out the canteen, the art room, and the best spot under the big gum tree for eating lunch. After school, Billy invited Albert to ride bikes around the neighbourhood. Billy listened when Albert talked and said kind things like, "It's okay to miss your old school. I'd miss mine too."

Albert felt calm and happy around Billy. He was like a green light shining, telling him it was safe to be himself.

Georgie was friendly too, but sometimes she was a bit tricky to understand. She helped Albert in class and shared her pencils, but when other friends came over, she'd say quietly, "Don't sit next to me today. They get jealous."

Albert liked Georgie, but sometimes he left their conversations feeling uncertain. A little like when you're waiting at an amber light, your parents might not be sure whether to stop or go. He decided to stay kind but be careful, giving Georgie space on days when she seemed unsure herself.

Then there was Max. At first, he seemed fun, and he reminded him of some of his old school friends. He was loud and full of jokes. He had lots of energy, and Albert quickly felt connected to him, even becoming a little braver, because Max did all the talking, and he could follow. It didn't take long for Albert to start to have mixed feelings about Max. He noticed Max laughed at people, not with them. The teacher always looked a bit tense when Max ran around the classroom.

"Why do you still talk about your old school?" Max teased. "You're here now. Get over it."

Max made up rules in games so he could win, and sometimes ignored Albert completely. When Albert told him, "That hurt my feelings," Max just shrugged.

After spending time with Max, Albert felt small inside, as if his heart were stuck at a red light.

That afternoon, Albert walked home alone. He stopped at the first crossing just as it turned amber. He didn't have the energy or the thinking to decide whether he had time to cross before it turned red. As he stared at the red light, he felt a growing sense of discomfort and impatience. He was desperate to get home to his family and see his baby sister; she always made him laugh. The green light went and made that lovely, safe sound that always felt good to hear. As Albert crossed, he began to see his new friends in much the same way as traffic lights. "Billy's green (he's kind and fair). Georgie's amber (she's nice most of the time, but confusing sometimes). Max is red (he's not safe for my heart right now)." Albert felt relieved that he could understand all the mixed feelings that had tired him all day. His last school had lots of red, green, and amber friends, and so did his football team. He guessed this was just how it had to be while everyone learned how to be their best.

As he crossed the next set, he was proud of himself and couldn't wait to tell his Mum all about it. There she was, waiting with her baby sister, who squealed with laughter and called out, "Abbott Abbott." He never wanted to forget how cute the sound of her voice trying to say his name was. Albert's Mum listened to every word Albert had to say about red, green, and amber light friends. She was so proud. "You're so wise, darling. Choose the friends who make you feel like you can go, not the ones who make you want to stop. Find the green light friends because that's exactly what you are."

Albert grinned. "Then I think I'll ride bikes with Billy again tomorrow."

And from that day on, Albert looked for the green lights in people, those who made his heart feel bright, brave, and free. He even made some amber light friends along the way, but always moved with caution.

Educators and parents

How do you know if a child has the traits of a red, amber, or green light friend?

How self-aware do you think most students are about being red, amber, or green light friends?

Do you think red and amber light traits tend to lead to more schoolyard conflict from your experience?

Do you think children tend to gravitate toward others with similar tendencies? In other words, do green light children tend to seek out other green light children?

Students

How do you think Albert felt when he had to move to a new school?

What helped Albert feel brave on his first day?

What did Billy, Georgie, and Max each do that showed the kind of friends they were? What did they do that was red, amber, and green?

Which friend would you most like to have? Why?

How did Albert's feelings change throughout the story?

Teaching and modelling the skill. Understanding traffic light friends (Self-Awareness, Communication Skills)

Some students may see themselves in the less likeable characters and feel embarrassed. Show compassion—every child is doing the best they can with the skills and support they have (Champlin, 2020).

When I read stories like Albert's in a classroom, students tend to look around and make eye contact with students they categorise as having certain personality types, almost as a bid to check that they are aware they are hurting others. This can also be challenging for students who are struggling socially.

Children who struggle are often aware of their behaviour, but personal or neurobiological factors can cause repeated mistakes (Champlin, 2020).

Model kindness and compassion. Children with red-light behaviours are not bad; they need help developing their skills. Everyone wants to belong. We can set boundaries and expectations, but we all contribute to a positive environment (Eisenberg et al., 2002).

Here's a tale of three friends, each shining with a different light. Listen closely—can you spot who's green, amber, or red? Maybe you'll recognise a bit of yourself in each character!

Once, there were three friends who were all very different. There was a **Green light, Grace**, an **Amber light, Alex**, and a **Red light, Jade**. They all liked playing on the oval.

Green light, Grace

Grace was a **Green Light Friend**. When someone fell over, she stopped her game and asked, "Are you okay? Do you want me to help you up?" Grace liked to include everyone. If she saw someone sitting alone, she'd wave and say, "Come play with us!" She also had the clever knack of always looking for something good in everyone. She liked something about everyone, even the red-light friends. Everyone liked Grace and felt safe around her.

Sometimes, Grace didn't get her way, and like everyone else, she felt annoyed. Sometimes, people were mean to Grace on purpose about her hardest challenge, learning. It never came easily to her. Grace never let this ruin someone else's day. Her parents taught her early about the power of our words, and she spoke with fairness and kindness. When angry, she took a few breaths before speaking. Grace spoke kindly even when things felt unfair. She would say, "I wanted to be 'it' today, but you can go first." "Are you okay? What you said was mean -I didn't think you were the kind of person that would be mean on purpose?"

After being with Grace, people felt **safe, happy, and calm**, like the warm sun on their face.

Amber light, Alex

Then there was **Amber light, Alex**. Alex was kind *sometimes*. He made everyone laugh, shared his snacks, but sometimes, he'd roll his eyes or say, "That's a baby game. You need to grow up!" Alex whispered secrets to one friend, leaving the others out. He didn't plan to hurt feelings; he just didn't notice when he did. When someone told him, "That made me sad," he'd usually pause and say, "Oh… I didn't realise. Sorry."

After playing with Alex, people felt a **mix of good and not-so-good** feelings, a little like the sky when the sun and rain come out at the same time.

Red light, Jade

Then there was **Red Light, Jade**. Jade could be fun, but only if things went *their* way. If someone disagreed, Jade would shout, "Fine! I didn't want to play with you anyway!" Jade sometimes called people names or made up rules that weren't fair. When someone told Jade to stop, Jade crossed their arms and said, "You're being a baby." After being with Jade, people often felt tired, worried, or small inside.

One day, the teacher asked everyone to draw a "friendship traffic light." Grace drew a big green circle and wrote, "Kind, fair, includes others." Alex drew an amber one and said, "Tries to be kind, but still learning." Jade looked at their red light and frowned. The teacher smiled gently. "We all have a bit of green, amber, and red inside us. What matters is noticing our colour and trying to move towards green." Their teacher always knew what to say to make everyone feel better.

Jade thought about that. At lunch, Jade noticed someone sitting alone and said quietly,

"Hey… do you want to join our game?" The person's face lit up. "Yes, please!" Grace smiled. "Look! Jade's turning green!" Everyone laughed and played together until the bell rang.

From that day on, the children learned to notice the colours of friendship, to spend more time with the greens, be kind but careful with the ambers, and use strong, calm words with the reds.

> **Group discussion questions**
> What do you think a green light friend is?
> What are some green light words a friend might say?
> What might make someone an amber light friend?
> Can you think of times when you've been an amber light friend (kind, but maybe not all the time)?
> What are some red-light behaviours that make friendships feel unsafe or unkind?
> Why is it important to notice how you feel inside when you're with a friend, like a traffic light in your heart?

Shine your friendship lights! (Self-Awareness)

Now that students understand friendship behaviours, expand self-awareness by helping them reflect on their own experiences (Yong, 2008).

Have students write or draw their own traffic lights, reflecting on their green, amber, and red behaviours. Remind them about self-compassion and that everyone is learning (Champlin, 2020).

> What are my green light behaviours? When do I show these the most?
> What are my amber light behaviours? When do I show these the most?
> What are my red-light behaviours? When do I show these the most?

Remind students we all have all the colours in us, and our goal is to keep moving towards green, learning from mistakes (Eisenberg et al., 2002; Rose & Rudolph, 2006).

Game time: Stop, slow down, or go? The friendship traffic lights game!

After self-reflection, have students move outside to release their emotions. Students act out red, amber, or green scenarios, responding by stopping (red), slowing (amber), or going (green) (Jones & Rutland, 2019).

Here are some scenarios to help:

Your friend listens to your story and smiles at you.
Green (kind and caring behaviour).

Your friend rolls their eyes when you make a mistake.
Red (unkind and disrespectful).

Your friend says sorry after accidentally bumping into you.
Green (thoughtful and respectful).
Your friend sometimes interrupts you when you're talking, then says, "Sorry, you go."
Amber (not perfect but trying to make it right).

Your friend ignores you when you ask to play and walks away.
Red (hurtful and unfriendly).

Your friend congratulates you when you win a game.
Green (supportive and positive).

Your friend tells you they don't want to play your game, but offers a kind reason and suggests an alternative.
Amber (honest and fair but needs balance).

Your friend talks about you behind your back.
Red (untrustworthy behaviour).

Your friend keeps your secret and checks if you're okay.
Green (trustworthy and caring).

Your friend sometimes leaves you out but invites you the next time.
Amber (mixed behaviour; needs reflection).

Your friend tells you the truth, even though it might hurt a little.
Amber (honest but could be handled gently).

Your friend cheers for you when you do well and claps for others, too.
Green (supportive, fair, and kind).

Your friend keeps checking your messages but doesn't reply.
Amber (confusing; might need a calm chat to check in).

Your friend shares your private story with others for a laugh.
Red (breaks trust).

Your friend admits they were wrong and tries to rectify the situation.
Green (takes responsibility and values the friendship).

Your friend makes jokes that put you down, then says, "It's just a joke."
Red (dismissive and hurtful, even if they don't mean to be).

Your friend helps you when you're upset, but expects you to help them every time they are.
Amber (caring but a bit one-sided).

Your friend listens to your opinion even when they disagree.
Green (respectful and emotionally mature).

Your friend only wants to hang out when it suits them.
Red (self-centred and unreliable).

Your friend teases you sometimes, but stops when you say it's not funny.
Amber (learning to respect boundaries).

Celebrate the learning with your students! Remind them: "We shine brightest together." Every day is a chance to be a green-light friend and help your classmates do the same.

What lights surround you? (Social Awareness, Empathy and Perspective Taking, Self-Awareness)

Young people know who feels safe, but sometimes adapt to fit in. Red and amber friends can seem fun, making it tricky to choose green-light friends (Jones & Rutland, 2019).

Group discussion

Ask the following questions and record the answers on the whiteboard to help students with the Role-Plays that follow.

1. How can you tell when a friend makes your heart feel "green"?
2. What can you do if someone with "red light" behaviour is also really nice to you and fun to be around?
3. What could help a friend with an amber light turn green?
4. What are some kind ways to set boundaries with an amber or red-light friend? (e.g., "I don't like it when you say that." "I still want to be friends, but not when you play that way." "I'm going to play somewhere else right now."
5. Is it possible for someone to show all three colours? If it were, how would you know what to do?

Personal reflection on friends to deepen individual awareness

Find a spot for students to lie on the grass or floor. Provide the following guidance, slowly and compassionately: *"Students, close your eyes and think about who's in your friendship circle at school (and outside of school). Who we spend our time with and focus our energy on can make a big difference in how we show up in the world. Friendships should uplift you and help you grow, not hold you back and drain you. Thinking about the people you are friends with who are green? Who is Amber? Who is red? Who is a bit of everything? Keep your heart and mind open. How can you hold hope for your red-light friends to learn and grow into green-light friends? How can you help your amber friends spend more effort on green light behaviour? How can you spend more time and uplift your green light friends?"*

Role plays

By now, your students have had plenty of role-play experience and should be able to come up with their own role plays. Another idea is to create a whole-class play based on Albert's story or the Traffic Light Friends story and perform it at an assembly or film it for parents and carers. Feel free to upload and share your brilliance at @thefriendshipblueprint.

Allow your students time to create short scenes illustrating green, amber, and red-light behaviours, then discuss what each feels like and what could make the situation greener.

Green light, GO! Remember: We're all in this friendship journey together

End with compassion: we all contribute to a positive school culture by showing green-light behaviours and supporting others in their growth (Eisenberg et al., 2002).

Gut feelings and friendship lights (Self-Awareness, Empathy, and Perspective Taking)

Often, we can sense that something is or isn't right in a friendship, but we can't quite put our finger on it. Some of us are excellent at tuning into our feelings but ignore them; others tune in and act, while still others push aside their gut feelings and don't act. Gut feelings are usually a sign to pay attention and listen. Gut feelings are our body's way of telling us something is not right.

Your friendship lights

Explain the concept of a friendship light within, a signal that helps you know how safe and happy a friendship feels. Just as there are green, amber, and red friendships, there are lights that illuminate within us when we observe those behaviours around us. Our "friendship light" comes from our gut feeling, and it's your body's way of helping you choose friends who make you feel happy and safe. It comes from our ancestors, with our survival brain activating it. The more you notice your lights, the better you get at finding friends who are good for you. If you tend to be a "worrier," your lights might be activated more than necessary; do some fact-checking to make sure it's accurate and not overthinking.

Green light within: Everything is going smoothly. You feel happy, safe, and comfortable around this friend. Your body feels relaxed and excited to spend time with them. Green light friends are kind, caring, and a lot of fun to be around.

Amber light within: This is a warning light. Your body might feel a bit nervous or unsure. Maybe your friend sometimes makes you feel upset or confused. Amber light means slow down, pay attention, and see if things improve before you spend too much time together.

Red light within: This is a stoplight. Your body feels tense, uncomfortable, or worried around this person. Red light friends might hurt your feelings or make you feel unsafe. It's okay to step back and take care of yourself.

Friendship light practice: Tuning into your gut feelings

Explain how you're about to facilitate an activity to explore gut feelings. Reinforce that everyone has a green, amber, and red light inside their body that helps them gauge their feelings about friends, and it can be very helpful to tune in and pay attention to these emotions. Sitting or lying down with eyes closed, ask the following questions:

Green light gut feelings

"Can you remember a time when you felt super happy with a friend? That's your green light. How did your body feel? Where were you? What was happening?"

Amber light gut feelings

"Now, think of a time a friend did something that made you a little unsure or worried. That's an amber light. What did your body feel like? Where were you? What was happening?"

Red light gut feelings

"Finally, think of a time a friend made you feel unsafe or really upset. That's a red light. What did your body feel like? Where were you? What was happening?"

Tuning in: Ask your students, "Next time you meet a new friend or play with your friends, notice your lights. If your body feels at ease, that's wonderful; this is probably an excellent friendship. If your body feels amber, remember to move forward carefully. Slow down, pay attention, keep an eye out for that red light. If your body feels red, stop, and protect yourself. Move towards the green light, people, and always remember that someone is there to help you. Don't keep your worries inside; adults can help."

> **Student reflection**
> "Why is it helpful to notice your friendship lights?"
> "Your friendship lights are your superpower. They help you find friends who make you feel safe, happy, and cared for. Do you think you're using yours enough?"

Friendship light role plays: Something doesn't seem right

Allow your students to come up with scenarios in which someone may appear friendly but, for some reason, makes them feel uncomfortable. Have fun exploring how people and situations can present themselves, and consider various solutions that are kind and constructive. Allow them to use inspiration from the characters in the stories so far, if they are struggling to come up with their own.

What is relational energy, and how are people like sunflowers? (Empathy and Perspective Taking, Communication Skills)

Relational energy is the feelings and energy we produce when interacting with others. You've probably heard the saying, "people won't always remember what you said or did, but they will always remember how you made them feel." Feelings are contagious. One element of having a survival brain is that we're wired to notice other people's moods and relational energy. We're wired to feel safer with people whose relational energy represents the green-light actions we've been exploring, rather than the red-light ones, where our bodies, on a neurobiological level, send signals that we're in danger. Spending time with red light relational energy, without the buffer of more green light relational energy and stress management tools, can push our bodies into survival mode more than is healthy.

Often, we pick up on people's relational energy in the first few moments of meeting. That feeling may grow, shrink, or remain the same. It's nothing personal; they may well be fantastic people, but something about them and the way they interact feels draining for you. We can't like everyone, and not everyone will like us. Our relational energy can also change with our age, circumstances, neurobiological hardwiring, and mood. Even the most uplifting person will have days when their relational energy may be flat or even draining.

Just like sunflowers turn towards the sunlight to grow stronger with the sun's energy, people turn towards other people as part of our biological need for safe and positive social connections. We can be uplifted or drained, depending on the kind of "relational energy" someone carries. Relational energy can change through the ups and downs of life, but most of the time, the feeling you get from another person stays similar. Relational energy comes from our character, values, and actions. People with healthy relational energy feel secure and safe in their relationships with others. They are usually trustworthy and kind. They show you, through their words and actions, that you're welcome and you belong. When they make social mistakes (and the truth be known, everyone does), it might feel surprising, because it's not how they usually behave. While good friends can sometimes say or do things that are unkind, safe friends with friendly relational energy don't make these mistakes intentionally or often, and when they do, they make amends.

Relational energy holds clues about a person's red, amber, and green friendship lights.

To strengthen student knowledge, share the 'Red, amber or green light relational energy?" poster (Figure 4.1).

Be a sunflower

Continuing the concept of relational energy and green light friendships being like the sun to a sunflower, ask students, "Have you ever felt happy or safe just being around someone? Or maybe a bit uneasy with someone else? That feeling is *relational energy*. People's energy can feel like green lights (safe and friendly), amber lights (sometimes tricky), or red lights (draining or

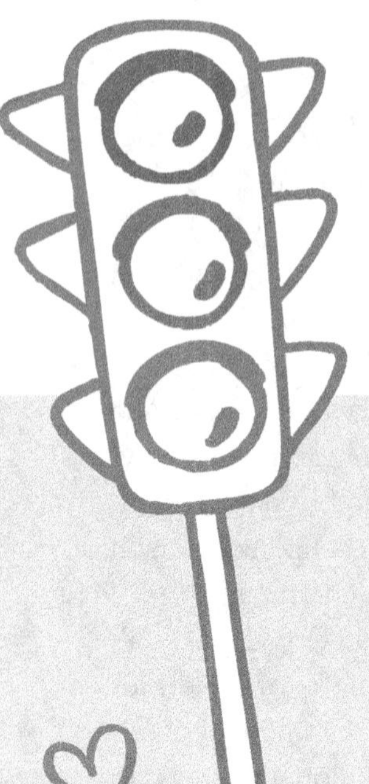

FRIENDSHIP TRAFFIC LIGHT
GREEN, AMBER, OR RED.

AMBER LIGHT
SLOW DOWN

This friendship can be kind or unkind. Try to make it better together.

- Inconsistent: kind and unkind
- Blames others
- Doesn't take no for an answer
- Sometimes includes, sometimes excludes
- Breaks promises

GREEN LIGHT
GO

This friendship is kind, fun, and safe. Keep it up.

- Kind
- Inclusive
- Honest and trustworthy
- Compassionate and empathetic
- Warm and friendly
- Helpful
- Respects boundaries, takes no for an answer.
- Genuine and loyal
- Keeps their word
- Accepts everyone, no judgment
- Cares about privacy
- Respects your time, energy, and boundaries
- Listens as much as talks
- Encouraging and supportive
- Consistent (you know what to expect).

RED LIGHT
STOP

This friendship feels hurtful. Tell a trusted adult and keep yourself safe.

- Mean on purpose
- Leaves others out
- Lies, even if it hurts others
- Shares private information
- Talks behind people's backs
- Judges and criticises others. (If they talk about others, they'll talk about you; don't get involved.)
- Won't compromise, wants everything their way.
- Emotionally draining
- Gives silent treatment or hurts you for setting boundaries

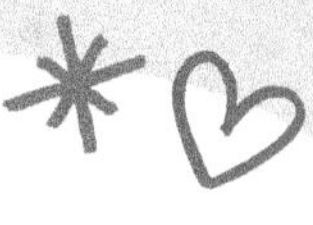

uncomfortable). Just like sunflowers turn towards the sun to grow, we turn towards people with good energy because it helps us feel safe and happy."

Sunflower rise

Once more, compare sunflowers turning towards the light, as people turn towards green light relational energy.

Call out the scenarios from the earlier green, red, and amber light relational energy examples. When the behaviour is green, students stand up and hold their hands high towards the sun (if outside) or the light (when indoors). When the behaviour is red or amber, students shrink by squatting for amber or sitting all the way on the ground for red.

Following the game, highlight that just like the sun helps sunflowers grow, their energy can help friends feel safe and happy.

Reflection

Ask your students:

"What is something you can do today to give green light relational energy to others?"

Key points:
Relational energy is contagious. Your energy affects others.
Green light energy is safe, kind, and uplifting.
People turn towards positive energy, like sunflowers towards sunlight.

We can all take responsibility for choosing kindness and giving off as much positive energy as possible ourselves. If we're having a bad day or struggle to show our green light energy skills, just let people know. In the Friendship Blueprint Community, no one is judged, and everyone feels safe and connected. Everyone belongs.

Game: Energy tag; green, amber, red

Find a space where everyone can move about easily.
Assign roles (informally, no props).
Explain, "Everyone is a 'sunflower' who can feel and give energy."

Select a student to serve as the "energy leader" to begin.

Refresh everyone's memory about green, amber, and red light energy.

Green energy: Friendly, safe, kind, makes others feel good.

Amber energy: Mixed, sometimes nice, sometimes unsure, or confusing.

Red energy: Unfriendly, draining, makes people feel uneasy.

Round 1: Walk and notice

Students walk slowly around the space.

The "energy leader" calls out "Green energy," "Amber energy," or "Red energy."

When students hear the word "green," they walk towards someone who emits friendly energy (smile, open posture).

When they hear red, they pause, take a step back, or shield themselves (like amber caution).

Round 2: Give green energy

Everyone walks around again.

This time, the goal is to provide green energy to at least two people by engaging in a friendly behaviour from the green light list earlier. Ask students to try their best to tune into how it feels when they *receive* green energy.

Round 3: Tag twist

One child (or the facilitator) is designated as the "Red Energy" (tagger).

Everyone else must move around and turn towards green energy from friends to be "safe zones." If a green energy friend gets tagged, they freeze until another friend gives them a green energy "boost" by doing something kind and friendly to unfreeze them.

> **Reflection questions**
>
> "How did it feel when you received green energy?"
>
> "What was it like giving green energy to someone?"
>
> "Could you notice red or amber energy from anyone? How did you respond?"
>
> "Like sunflowers, we turn towards energy that helps us grow. How can you be a green light for your friends today?"

Doc friendship and traffic light energy consolidation. (Conflict Resolution and Problem Solving, Empathy, and Perspective Taking)

To further develop reflective thinking, empathy, and compassion, invite your students to write or draw about a fabricated friendship problem. Examples of a problem might be:

"Dear Doc Friendship, my friend is only friendly to me when we aren't at school. When we're at school, he ignores me. Is it okay if they are only nice to me in private?"

"Dear Doc Friendship, my friend always tells me what to do. Is that normal?"

"Dear Doc Friendship, my friend borrowed my remote-control car and broke it. They gave it back to me and acted as if nothing had happened. Should I say something?"

Students often enjoy games like this where they can explore the woes of friendship without needing to open up more than they are ready to or share personal worries and experiences. Once all the problems have been written or drawn, divide the students into pairs, equip them with recording equipment, and, if possible, add some costumes for fun. Allow students to take turns being "Doc Friendship" and invite them to do their best to help their "patient" understand whether they are experiencing a red, green, or amber friendship light. Then have them notice the energy in their bodies and work together to come up with a solution.

Role plays

Invite students to role-play the following scenarios, then allow the class to analyse it further using the discussion questions that follow.

> **1. Sharing private information**
> Marcus tells Liesl something private, and Liesl promises not to tell. The next day at school, everyone knows. When Marcus asks Liesl if she was the one who told everyone, she says, "It's no big deal, you're overreacting."

Red light (trust and boundaries disrespected).
How would you feel if you were Marcus?
Why is this a red light?
What would a green light response be instead?

2. ***Kind encourager***

Talia feels nervous before her class speech. Her friend Sam says, "You've got this. I'll sit at the front and smile at you!"

Green light (empathy and support shown).
How did Sam show they're a green light friend?
How would you feel if you had a friend like Sam?
What kind of friend do you want to be?

3. ***Hot and cold friend***

Marlo is nice some days, but on other days ignores you or rolls his eyes at your jokes.

Orange light (confusing and inconsistent).
What makes this an orange flag?
Why is it important to notice patterns in friendships?
What would you do if this kept happening?

4. ***Bossy buddy***

A friend always tells you what to do at recess: "Sit here! Play this! Don't talk to them."

Red light (power imbalance, controlling).
Is that how teamwork and choices in friendship should feel?
What's the difference between being a leader and being bossy?

5. ***Shared joy***

You win a prize in class. Your friend high-fives you and says, "I'm so proud of you!"

Green light (celebrates other people's success and happiness).
How does it feel to be supported like this?
How do green light friends react to your good news?

6. ***The guilt trip***

You can't hang out after school, and your friend says, "Wow, I guess you don't care about me anymore."

Orange light (emotional pressure, perspective).
How could this make someone feel?
What would be a more respectful way for a friend to respond?

7. *Active listener*

You're upset about something that happened at lunch. Your friend sits with you and says, "Tell me what happened, I'm here."

Green light (offering listening and emotional support).

What makes someone a good listener?

Why is this a green light moment?

8. *The blamer*

When something goes wrong in a group game, your friend always blames you (even when it isn't your fault).

Red light (unfair and irresponsible).

How would that feel over time?

What might this show you about their ability to take responsibility?

9. *Friend one day, gone the next*

Your friend is super nice when you're alone, but ignores you when other people are around.

Orange light (inconsistent with their behaviour towards you).

Why is this confusing?

What might be going on from their perspective?

Should a friend make you feel invisible?

10. *You can be you*

Other people have kept telling you that your favourite hobby is weird. Your friend says, "I know nothing about that, can I have a try? It looks interesting."

Green light (kindness, compassion, empathy, inclusion).

How does this kind of friendship help you feel safe to be yourself?

Why is that important?

Doc friendship's prescription for green light relational energy

Before beginning this last activity in this chapter, take a breath and a moment to remember being the same age your students are now. During primary school, mistakes are common, and we can help young people learn from them to improve and move forward, avoiding the intentional repetition of the same mistake. As a character is still developing in these early years, someone with red and amber friendship lights might also have many green lights and vice versa. This can be very confusing. Depending on which lights they show most, it can be tricky to tell if the person is a kind and safe friend to connect with.

Allow students some time to reflect on and discuss the following questions in small groups (or individually if they work better on their own).

> Ways to work out a solution when a friend is showing green, amber, and red lights.
> One thing I'll try this week to be a green friendship light is…
> If I make a mistake and turn on a red friendship light, I can make it better by…

Bring the discussion back to the class and invite students to create friendship goals based on their reflections. Try to check in regularly with students who struggle to apply social skills that connect with the green light skills. Provide plenty of positive feedback when they're meeting their friendship goals, and respond to their challenging moments with a warm, supportive approach.

It's important to remember how learning and growing involve mistakes and detours. Red lights are not labels; they are signals for reflection and possible support. Green lights suggest readiness for positive relationships, but even children who struggle can become great friends with the right guidance, patience, and modelling. Behaviour is always communication, and young people are doing the best they can with the skills and knowledge they have so far.

Encouraging young people to seek out friends who are kind, respectful, and emotionally supportive helps them develop lifelong skills for healthy relationships.

Key takeaways from Chapter 4: The red, green, and amber friendship lights

- Recognising and interpreting "traffic light" signals in friendships helps them identify safe (green), confusing (amber), and unsafe (red) behaviours.

- Self-awareness helps students to reflect on their own emotions and social roles within friendships. Empathy and perspective-taking are developed as students consider how their actions and words affect others.
- The conflict-resolution and problem-solving strategies introduced in this chapter empower students to handle disagreements positively by being a green-light friend.
- The traffic light model provides a practical framework for students to assess and respond to different friendship situations.
- All skills and activities are aligned with the Australian Curriculum's requirements for health and social-emotional wellbeing capabilities.

Call to action

Use the traffic light model daily and notice the colour of student friendships. Help students strive to be a "green light" friend and support others in developing positive relationship skills to foster a safer, more caring school community. Create a culture of green light friendships by encouraging peer mentoring, educator acknowledgement for their green light energy, parent support, as well as celebrating when students demonstrate the culture alive in their everyday interactions.

References

Champlin, B. (2020). *Development and importance of children's skills in emotional regulation essay example | Topics and well written essays - 2000 words - 1*. Studentshare. https://studentshare.org/psychology/1807572-consider-the-development-and-importance-of-childrens-skills-in-emotional-regulation#cite_document_box

Eisenberg, N., Guthrie, I. K., Cumberland, A., Murphy, B. C., Shepard, S. A., Zhou, Q., & Carlo, G. (2002). Prosocial development in early adulthood: a longitudinal study. *Journal of Personality and Social Psychology*, 82(6), 993–1006. https://pubmed.ncbi.nlm.nih.gov/12051585/

Jones, S. E., & Rutland, A. (2019). Children's social appraisal of exclusion in friendship groups. *International Journal of Bullying Prevention, 2*. https://doi.org/10.1007/s42380-019-00022-w

Rose, A. J., & Rudolph, K. D. (2006). A review of sex differences in peer relationship processes: Potential trade-offs for the emotional and behavioral development of girls and boys. *Psychological Bulletin, 132*(1), 98–131. https://doi.org/10.1037/0033-2909.132.1.98

Rubin, K. H., Bukowski, W. M., & Parker, J. G. (2006). Peer interactions, relationships, and groups. In N. Eisenberg (Ed.), *Handbook of Child Psychology* (6th ed., Vol. 3, pp. 571–645). John Wiley & Sons, Inc.
Yong, E. (2008). *Children learn to share by age 7–8. Science.* https://www.nationalgeographic.com/science/article/children-learn-to-share-by-age-7-8

Appendix: Super friendship toolbox and brilliant bonus ideas

1. Friendship traffic light poster: Print or draw your own, with fun icons or animal characters for each colour! Display in your classroom and at home.
2. Friendship detective journal: Write or draw about your friendship adventures: Who helped you feel green-light happy? Did you notice any amber or red? Add comic strips or short illustrated stories about your real-life scenarios.
3. Traffic light scenarios: Use the examples in the chapter for a fun class game or role-play. Try "Friendship Freeze Frames," where you act out and freeze on a traffic light colour for your classmates to guess.
4. Sunflower energy activity: Have your own Sunflower Rise game outside or in the classroom! Make it even more fun by pairing it with art, draw or paint what a green-light friendship looks like.
5. Doc friendship letters: Write, record, or even perform your own advice letters and skits to help solve tricky friendship problems. Use costumes and props to make it memorable!
6. Green light goals chart: Make a chart to track your green-light behaviours each week. Celebrate progress with stickers, badges, or a special "Green Light Day!"
7. Reflection questions: Use the questions from the chapter to check in with your feelings and friendship lights. Finish each session with a Friendship Cheer or affirmation!
8. Friendship bracelets: Make bracelets using green, amber, and red beads to help you remember the lessons and talk about your feelings.
9. Take-home family challenge: Bring the traffic light guide home and teach your family how to use the friendship lights language. Draw or write about a green-light moment at home.

10. Friendship songs and chants: Create or learn simple songs and chants to help everyone remember what each light means and encourage green-light actions every day.
11. Friendship star board: Add a star for every green-light action in your class. Watch the board fill up and celebrate together!

Remember: Every day is a new chance to shine your green light! Try out your Friendship Detective skills every day! Notice which colour your friendships are—are you helping to make your school a place full of green lights? Celebrate every time you show green-light behaviours, and cheer on friends who do the same. Together, let's make our classrooms the happiest, kindest places to be!

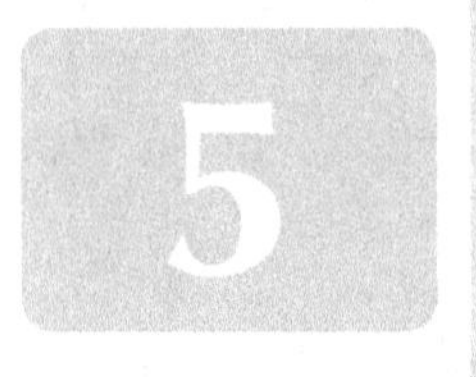

Friendly communication for strong and healthy friendships

While communication styles naturally vary, schools can strengthen their culture, by teaching and encouraging a shared language of mutually respectful communication that breaks down barriers and improves connections

Nelson Mandela reminded us that forgiveness or at the very least, moving forward without ruminating on past hurts, is much healthier than resentment, by coining the phrase, "Resentment is like drinking poison and then hoping it will kill your enemies."

The great friendship communication quest!

Welcome, brave adventurers! In this chapter, you're about to set off on a quest to become Friendship Communication Champions. Along the way, you'll collect special skills and magical habits that help you build strong, happy friendships. Get ready for games, challenges, and secret missions that make learning about talking and listening fun, friendly, and full of surprises!

Communication is friendship in action (Liu, 2018). The way you talk, listen, and even stand can help build bridges to new friends or create walls that keep people out. Every child is a unique communicator—some

DOI: 10.4324/9781003617570-5

are quiet, some love to talk, and some use their faces or hands more than words! This chapter is packed with fun activities, real-life stories, and games to help you find your voice, listen with your heart, and make every friendship sparkle.

You'll discover superpowers like active listening (that means really paying attention!), giving genuine compliments, asking for help, setting boundaries, and staying cool when things get tricky. Through role-play, games, and team quests, you'll practice kindness and learn to be a communication superstar!

Setting the scene: Welcome to friendship island (Overview: Self-Awareness, Communication, Empathy, Conflict Resolution)

Imagine your classroom is a big, bright island. Sometimes the sun shines, and everyone gets along. Other times, stormy clouds (disagreements!) roll in. Here, you'll learn how to use your communication skills as your "weather tools" to bring back the sunshine and help everyone feel welcome. It's normal for friends to disagree or test each other's limits—just like the changing weather! That's how you practice real-life friendship skills. School and home are your practice fields for these important life skills. When emotions run high, sometimes kindness takes a nap—especially in disagreements between friends or siblings! But don't worry, you'll learn how to wake kindness up and keep it working, even when feelings are strong. Friendly communication is like glue that holds friendships together. It helps your friends feel important, safe, and happy to share what's on their minds. Skills like active listening, empathy, and positive body language are your secret ingredients for making every friendship feel safe, special, and full of care. Great friendships are like see-saws—they work best when everyone gets a turn! Taking turns talking and listening helps everyone feel respected and understood. Friendly communication makes boundaries clear and helps friendships grow stronger. This chapter is your toolkit for becoming a Friendship Communication Champion—full of tips, stories, and games for everyone, no matter how you like to communicate.

Spotting the skill (Observation & Reflection) (Self-Awareness, Empathy and Perspective Taking, Communication Skills)

Let's dive into a real-life friendship story to see how different communication styles can affect how we feel and connect. Read this case study to your students

Winter and Summer were friends as different as the seasons they were named after.

Winter liked quiet and routine; Summer enjoyed noise and people. Winter preferred one-on-one time, while Summer wanted Winter to join her with other friends.

Despite their differences, they cared deeply for each other.

Summer would run over, shouting, "Winter, let's jump on the trampoline with everyone!" The loudness startled Winter, who didn't like noise. "You scared me," she'd say. Summer rolled her eyes, "You're so serious!" The sharp tone and eye roll hurt. Winter thought, "Why can't I be more like Summer?"

Summer left to join her friends. Later, Winter avoided Summer, who asked, "Why are you so grumpy?"

Winter whispered, "I'm not grumpy. I just feel like you don't listen."

Summer huffed and left, not realising their faces, tones, and body language spoke louder than words.

By the last school bell, the girls were both very upset.

The teacher reminded them to choose kindness and respect differences (Culver, 2024; Neff, 2011). Words and actions can't be undone. **He** encouraged reflection and repair.

They went home separately, cried with their families, and felt heavy-hearted.

After a good night's sleep and a little break from each other, both their minds were clear. Words weren't needed. Their eyes, the warmth from their hearts, and their outstretched hands spoke a thousand words.

They realised neither way of being was better. Quiet and noise both matter. Kindness, spoken or not, can heal misunderstandings.

Educator reflection questions

How self-aware do you think your students are about their nonverbal and verbal communication?

Do they tend to be stronger in one or the other?

What has been the best way you've learnt so far to teach these skills to your students?

What makes it hard for them to learn these skills from your experience?

Student reflection

What was complicated about this friendship?

How do you think they will move forward to make things go smoothly in the future?

What could each of them learn from the other?

Can you think of a friend you like a lot and who you're also very different from? What could you learn from them?

Making communication feel like a green light

Verbal and nonverbal cues shape relationships and a sense of belonging (Goleman, 1995; Kennedy-Moore & Mclaughlin, 2017; Liu, 2018; Neff, 2011). Skills vary, especially for neurodivergent individuals and across cultures.

Teach students to respect diversity and practice self-leadership in communication (Neff, 2011; UNESCO, 2022).

Friendly vs. unfriendly game

Select a confident student to role-play a conversation with you. You'll model poor communication; they'll model the best. Check they're ready for the challenge.

Their goal: discuss weekend plans. Your goal: break the rules of friendly communication.

Show and review the 'Communication Blueprint' poster together.

During the mock conversation, students stand for friendly skills and sit for unfriendly ones. Watch for nonverbal cues (Figure 5.1).

KIND COMMUNICATION

USE SIMPLE, KIND WORDS, AND HAVE FUN.

- ▶ Listen with your eyes and ears. Let friends finish before you talk.
- ▶ Use kind, clear words. "Please," "thank you," and compliments make friends smile.
- ▶ Take turns. Share the conversation.
- ▶ Ask questions like "How?" or "Why?" to keep the chat going.
- ▶ Only joke if everyone is happy. Laugh with, not at others. Not sure? Ask an adult.
- ▶ Show kindness in your body language, smile, relax, and give people space.
- ▶ Match your voice to how others feel. Be gentle for comfort, excited for good news.
- ▶ Wait your turn to speak. Everyone likes to be heard.

BODY LANGUAGE: ACTIONS SPEAK LOUDER THAN WORDS.

- ▶ Look and listen. Nodding shows you care, even if eye contact is hard.
- ▶ Relax your body. Smile and use friendly faces.
- ▶ Give friends space. Don't stand too close or touch if it's not comfortable.
- ▶ Match your voice to the mood. Use a calm voice for comfort and an excited one for good news.
- ▶ Wait your turn to talk. Patience and respect make everyone feel good.

SMALL ACTIONS MATTER. BE KIND WITH YOUR BODY LANGUAGE.

KIND WORDS AND ACTIONS BUILD STRONG FRIENDSHIPS. BE KIND, BE RESPECTFUL, AND KEEP LEARNING TOGETHER.

Active listening detective game

Active listening can be challenging at all ages, especially for those who are shy and anxious. Some become fixated on how to respond and what to say next, and can't give their full attention to the person speaking to them. This can make them appear aloof and unsupportive, potentially fracturing a friendship that was on the verge of developing.

Review the poster again after completing the mock conversation game.

Choose a speaker to tell a 30–60 second story using a timer.

Listeners become detectives

While the speaker talks, the rest of the group are "Listening Detectives." Their job is to *show* they are listening by:

Looking in the speaker's direction.
Using eye contact if they feel comfortable.
Nodding sometimes.
Waiting without interrupting.
Matching their facial expression to the story (or letting the group know if that's hard for them).

Detective check-in

After the speaker finishes, the "Listening Detectives" take turns saying one detail they remember from the story.
The speaker can give a "thumbs up" if the listener remembered correctly.
Switch Roles. A new speaker is chosen, and the game repeats until everyone has had a chance to speak.

Listening detectives pair play

Divide your class into pairs where each partner tells a story, and the other must retell it in 2–3 sentences. The more your students practice being deliberate with their active listening skills through games like these, the more natural and comfortable it will become.

Listening Detective Checklist

Name: ______________________________

Did I…

1. Look towards the speaker (face or body turned towards them)?
   ☐ Yes   ☐ No
2. Use eye contact (if I feel comfortable)?
   ☐ Yes   ☐ No
3. Let others know eye contact is tricky for me.
   ☐ Yes   ☐ No
4. Nod sometimes to show I'm listening?
   ☐ Yes   ☐ No
5. Wait my turn (didn't interrupt until they finished)?
   ☐ Yes   ☐ No
6. Match my face to the story (smile if happy, look surprised if shocking, etc.)?
   ☐ Yes   ☐ No
7. Let them know my face isn't very expressive, but I was listening.
   ☐ Yes   ☐ No
8. Remember something from the story?
   ☐ Yes   ☐ No

   (If yes, what did I remember? ______________________)

Role plays to practice active listening for green light communication

Divide the class into pairs, ready to role-play the following scenarios that focus on active listening:

The birthday party plan

Roles: Planner, Listener

Scenario: One child explains how they want their birthday party (theme, cake, games). The listener repeats back the key ideas to show they were listening.

The lost puppy

Roles: Child who lost a puppy, Helper

Scenario: The child describes the puppy (colour, size, collar, and last seen location). The listener repeats the description and asks a clarifying question.

My weekend adventure

Roles: Storyteller, Listener

Scenario: The storyteller shares something fun they did over the weekend. The listener shows they are engaged by nodding, keeping eye contact, and asking one curious question.

The shopping list

Roles: Shopper, Listener

Scenario: The shopper tells the listener what they need to buy (e.g., apples, bread, milk). The listener repeats the list back correctly.

The secret instructions

Roles: Instruction Giver, Follower

Scenario: The instructor explains how to draw a simple picture (a house, a tree, or a smiley face) without showing it. The listener follows the directions carefully.

The friendship problem

Roles: Child with a problem, Listener

Scenario: One child explains a friendship problem (e.g., someone didn't share, someone cut in line). The listener shows empathy by saying, "That sounds…" or "I understand…"

The new game rules

Roles: Game Explainer, Listener

Scenario: One child explains the rules of a new game. The listener listens carefully, then tries to explain the rules back.

The class helper

Roles: Teacher giving directions, Class Helper listening
Scenario: The "teacher" gives instructions for helping (e.g., "Can you hand out the pencils, then collect the books, then put the markers away?"). The listener repeats back before starting.

Shining a light on friendly nonverbal communication, a discussion

Start by asking your students, "Have you ever noticed how someone's mood and facial expressions can change your mood?" Give an example of a time you were happily minding your own business, and someone dumped all their grumpiness on you, and you felt emotionally uprooted. Now ask them to think of a time when they went somewhere and were greeted by a warm, friendly face. How did that feel? Did it lift their mood?

We have so much power in what we choose to say and do. For children who tend to have flat facial expressions, acknowledge that this is a normal and healthy variation and point out that their facial expressions may not accurately reflect their emotions. Ask, "What other ways can you show friendliness without using your face and words?"

Game: charades

Invite volunteers to act out the following scenarios without using words, relying solely on nonverbal communication.

Lost something

Act out losing something important and looking everywhere for it.

Line cutter

Show that someone cut in front of you in line, and you don't know what to do.

Excited wave

Act out seeing a friend across the playground and trying to get their attention.

Want to join in

Show that you want to join a game but feel too nervous to ask.

Feeling left out

Act out feeling sad while others are laughing together without you.

Need help

Show that you're struggling to lift or move something heavy and that you want help.

Proud moment

Act out being really happy because you solved something tricky or did a great job.

Oops, sorry!

Act out bumping into someone and showing that you feel sorry for them.

Cheering up a friend

Act out making silly faces or showing kindness to make a sad friend feel better.

Active listener

Act out listening carefully and showing interest in what someone is saying.

Nonverbal communication game: Guess what I'm feeling 123

Divide the group into pairs and let them practice their facial expressions together for three emotions. Simplify the first round with "angry, happy, and sad." On go, the students stand back-to-back and decide which emotion they will express when you count to three and ask them to turn around. Prepare students to decide which expression they will reveal. For fun, they can imagine they are sending a message to their partner to express the same emotion. There will be three rounds per pair, and the goal is to synchronise as often as possible. On the count of three, students jump from back-to-back to face-to-face to reveal their chosen emotion. Watch the fun and connection as they connect through both getting it right and wrong.

Group discussion: The power of communication and our responsibility to be kind

Kindness is never wasted, and it's contagious. Intentional cruelty happens until a child is taught better and held accountable through a school culture with zero tolerance for intentional cruelty.

The most verbally and non-verbally expressive person in a room can quickly change the feeling in a space. If the social script in your school is to be kind, one child at a time, along with one educator at a time, can together change the culture into one of kindness.

Ask your students to imagine having a happy, friendly time at school, only for someone loud and mean to come in and shout at everyone. Then offer the following questions:

Do you think you could stay happy in this situation and keep doing what you were doing, or would your mood change?
Do you think it's fair to talk to others like this?
Is it everyone's responsibility to try to be kind?
Could a kind person do this?
What might be behind this kind of behaviour?

Nonverbal communication goal for friendly, green light communication

Invite students to write or draw about how they envision their character and values showing up in the world.
Do they want to show attributes like warmth, kindness, gentleness, fun, friendliness, patience, fairness, and understanding?
What would they gain for themselves and others if they did show those behaviours?
What might they lose for themselves and others if they were to do the opposite?

Support your students in setting a goal for how they want to show up when they walk through the school gates each morning. Share how you want to lead yourself to show up and take full responsibility to do what you can to show up this way.

Being deliberate and intentional about how our character shows up in the world is a powerful way to change behaviour and cultures for the better.

Words matter. The art of friendly verbal communication. (Communication Skills, Empathy and Perspective Taking, Conflict Resolution, and Problem Solving)

Children sometimes say or do things that hurt others—often without realising the impact (Kennedy-Moore & Mclaughlin, 2017). As adults, we must model responsible, kind communication and show how to make things right when mistakes happen.

Group discussion: The toothpaste tube and friendships

Invite the group to draw two toothpaste tubes, each taking up a page. Inside the first tube, ask them to fill it with words that are friendly and that they enjoy hearing others say to them. Younger students can draw the feelings and actions they love to experience from others. Inside the second toothpaste tube, they can fill it with words that hurt and drawings showing hurtful words and actions. Once students have completed their drawings, invite them to share their responses with a small group or the class.

Ask your students:

"Why do you think I asked you to put your words and drawings inside a toothpaste tube?"

Many students will have heard the analogy that once you squeeze toothpaste out of a tube, you can't push it back inside. Our words and actions are no different. Once they are out, we can't put them back into our hearts and minds. Whatever we say and do will elicit a response from others, and it's our responsibility to work hard to communicate and act in ways that aren't hurtful to others.

When their work is completed, display their pieces, and set the goal of working hard, being responsible for what we say and do, and remembering that we can all learn and grow our friendship skills. It's also essential to remember that not everyone has the same knowledge, skills, and experience; everyone is learning. Self-leadership means focusing on what we *can do* to be the best versions of ourselves.

Discussion: Which words build friendships and which harm them? (Culver, 2024)

Recording your answers on the whiteboard, with one side showing friendly words and the other showing unfriendly words, gives students ample time to consider their responses. Once they have finished their brainstorm, share the poster or project the image that follows to see how close they came to the words and language that neuroscientists have found helpful or unhelpful for friendships. Encourage them for coming up with their own (Figure 5.2).

Word energy catch and dodge game

To help children recognise how words and tone can make people feel, and to encourage friendly, inclusive, kind, and empathetic communication, prepare everyone for the game.

Ask: "If words had colours, what colour do you think kind words would be? What about mean words?"

Explain that every word gives off energy like green light (friendly), amber (unsure), or red light energy (hurtful).

The goal of the game is to give off green light words that help everyone feel included, safe, and valued.

Catch or dodge the words

Everyone stands in a circle.

The teacher calls out a word or phrase from the previous poster. Adjust the words to suit what your age group and school culture are comfortable with.

If the word feels friendly, kind, or inclusive, children pretend to catch it with both hands and say, "Got it!"
If the word feels unfriendly, mean, or exclusive, children dodge it (step to the side or duck) and say "No thanks!"

Pause after each word for a brief chat:

"Why did we catch that word?"
"Why did we dodge that one?"
"How might that word make someone feel?"

BLUEPRINT WORDS

FRIENDLY WORDS
BUILD FRIENDSHIPS

The words you choose can build or break a friendship.
Choose friendly words.

Use these
GREEN-LIGHT WORDS

Green words build trust and
help everyone feel included.

Hi • Please • Thank you • Excuse me
You're welcome • Want to join us? • Sorry
Can I help? • You're brave • Everyone's invited
How can I help? • That's okay • Try again
You can do it • I like your idea
Nice effort • I understand • You're awesome
You're good at that

AMBER WORDS

**Use carefully, they might
hurt someone's feelings.**

Amber words can sting. Try to use
green (friendly) words instead.

Whatever • That's weird
Overreacting • Not now • Don't care
Just kidding (after being mean)
Who cares? • No one cares
You're too sensitive

Never use
RED-LIGHT WORDS

Hurtful words are never okay.

Red words break trust and hurt
feelings. Always choose kind words.

You can't play • That's for boys/girls only
Weirdo • Dumb • Loser • Stupid • Ugly • Freak
Your skin's weird • You talk funny • Go away
I don't like you • That's gay • Boys don't cry
Sh#% up • You're not one of us • I hate you
We all hate you • You're not good enough

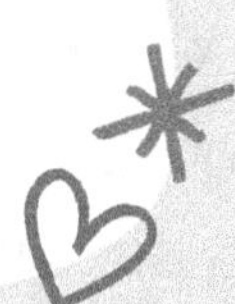
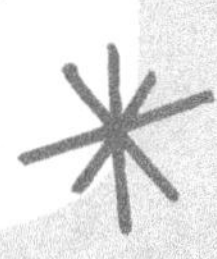

Discussion and reflection

"How do our words affect others?"

"Can you think of a time someone's words made you feel really good?"

"What could we say if we hear someone using a hurtful word?"

"What could we do if we say something by accident that hurts someone's feelings?"

Reinforce that everyone can make mistakes, but kind people repair with words like "I'm sorry," "I didn't mean to hurt you," or "Thanks for telling me."

Goal: word power challenge

Set a weekly goal for students to use five green-light words or sentences each day.

Conversation skills 101

Learning to be fair and balanced in a conversation is a powerful skill that can help everyone at home, at school, and at work. Divide your class into pairs and allow each pair 10 minutes to have a conversation using the following open-ended questions. They can take notes if they prefer, as they will be sharing three facts about their partner with the group afterwards.

How can people tell you don't like something?

What do you like most about yourself?

What's something that most people don't know about you?

Who is someone you wish you were still friends with but don't see anymore?

If you wrote a book, what would it be about?

What's something you wish you knew how to do and why?

If you could go back and fix a mistake you made, what would it be?

What could you teach another person your age?

What has been the hardest "first" for you? (first day of school, first day at a new sport, first friendship fight, first "no" for something you really wanted to hear, "yes" for?

What is most important for you in a friendship?

What is the kindest thing someone has ever done for you?

What's your favourite thing to do that doesn't cost money?

Describe something lucky that happened to you.

Invite students to share something they learned about their partner, doing their best to remember without notes. Be mindful that this may be difficult for some children, especially those with learning differences.

Reciprocity: Friendly communication is a two-way street. (Communication skills, Empathy, and Perspective Taking)

Primary school children often remain egocentric and may not have developed the ability to listen with consistent focus and concentration. Some either monopolise the conversation, fail to listen properly, or contribute more than their share. This is a skill everyone can improve, and the benefits include a deeper connection with others and enhanced social communication skills that can last a lifetime.

Taking turns, listening actively, and responding thoughtfully all help us build the friendly habit of reciprocal conversation.

Conversation circuit

Set up three or four "stations" in your classroom or space, and leave a prompt at each to let students know what to do when they reach that area.

Station 1: Mirror chat: Practice reflecting back what someone says (and add your own idea)

Children work in pairs.
Child A shares a short sentence about their day or a favourite thing. (e.g., "I had bacon and eggs for breakfast.")
Child B mirrors part of what was said and adds their own related idea. ("You had bacon and eggs for breakfast? I had cereal.")
Switch roles after each turn.
Encourage follow-up questions to deepen the exchange.

Station 2: Story pass: Build on each other's ideas and maintain a back-and-forth flow

Children sit in a circle.
Starts a story with one sentence (e.g., the dragon woke up ready for a day full of adventure).

Each child adds a sentence that connects to the previous one (e.g., his eyes
turned towards his little brother, and he knew just what to do).
Continue until everyone has contributed at least once.
Encourage creativity. Funny or imaginative ideas make it more engaging.

Station 3: Question chain: Practice asking and answering questions to keep a conversation going

Children sit or stand in a circle.
Child A asks a question to Child B.
Child B answers AND immediately asks another child a new question.
Keep the chain going around the circle.
Make questions light and playful to encourage participation.

Station 4: Bounce-back chat: Reinforce turn-taking and listening using a physical "conversation ball"

Children toss a soft ball to one another.
The catcher answers a short question or shares a thought, then tosses the
ball to someone else with a new question.
Emphasise polite listening cues, such as nodding, maintaining eye contact,
or repeating a key detail from the previous speaker.

Rotation and reflection

Children spend 5–7 minutes at each station. Alternatively, guide the
class through each station together if needed.

After completing all stations, gather for a reflection discussion:

"Which station was the most fun?"
"How did it feel when someone really listened to you?"
"What makes a conversation easy and friendly?"

Friendly communication role plays

Have students role-play in pairs. Afterwards, let them present to the group or
record their role-plays to share with families or other classes.

Rude exclusion role play

Unfriendly behaviour:

Child A is talking about their weekend plans, but **Child B** repeatedly interrupts and talks over them.

Child A feels ignored and frustrated, while **Child B** doesn't seem to notice.

Friendly communication solution:

Child A: "I know it's hard for you to listen, I just really want you to listen to something that matters to me.

Child B: "I'm sorry, I'll keep trying. Can we try again?

Interruption role play

Unfriendly behaviour:

Child A: "I'm going to the beach this weekend with my family. I'm so excited!"
Child B (interrupting): "I went to the park last weekend and saw a dog there. It was huge!"
Child A: "I was telling you about my weekend."
Child B: "Yeah, but I just wanted to share about the dog."

Friendly communication solution:

Child A (calmly): "I'd really like to tell you about my weekend first, then you can tell me about the dog. It's important to me that you listen when I'm speaking."
Child B (acknowledging): "Sorry, I didn't mean to interrupt. I'll wait for my turn to talk."
Child A: "Thanks! I can't wait to hear about the dog afterwards."

Active listening **and turn-taking** are key (Ryan & Deci, 2000).
Allow others to speak without interruption and express feelings calmly if interrupted.

Excluding a friend

Unfriendly behaviour:

Child A and **Child B** are playing a game together when **Child C** wants to join but is told, "You're not good at this game, just watch us play."

Child A: "Let's play tag. You're 'it'!"
Child B: "Yeah, we're good at this game, it'll be fun."
Child C: "Can I play too?"
Child A: "No, you're not good at tag. Just watch us."

Friendly communication solution:

Child C (feeling sad): "I feel left out when you say I can't play. Can I try? I'll do my best!"
Child A (realising): "Sorry, I didn't mean to make you feel bad. You can play with us! It's more fun when everyone plays anyway."
Child B: "Yeah, let's all play together. It'll be more fun that way!"

Honest feelings solve problems and build understanding (Neff, 2011).

Body language misunderstanding

Unfriendly behaviour:

Child A is speaking to **Child B**, but **Child B** is crossing their arms, rolling their eyes, and looking away, making **Child A** feel as though they aren't interested or are being rude.
Child A: "I wanted to tell you about the new book I got."
Child B (crossing arms, rolling eyes, looking away): "Uh-huh, sure."
Child A: "You don't seem to be listening. You look upset. Did I do something wrong?"
Child B: "No, I'm just tired."

Friendly communication solution:

Child A: "I didn't mean to make you feel like you had to listen. I'd like to share something exciting with you. If you're tired, we can talk later."
Child B (softening): "Sorry for making it seem like I wasn't interested. I was just feeling tired, but I'd love to hear about your book."
Child A: "Thanks for understanding! I'll tell you more when you feel ready."

Clear, respectful expression prevents misunderstandings (Kennedy-Moore & Mclaughlin, 2017).

Teasing and hurtful words

Unfriendly behaviour:

Child A makes fun of **Child B's** choice of clothes, calling them "weird" in front of others.
Child A: "Why are you wearing that? You look weird!"
Child B (feeling hurt): "Why would you say that?"
Child A: "It's just a joke. You don't need to get upset."
Child B: "It really hurt my feelings when you said that."

Friendly communication solution:

Child A (realising): "I'm sorry, I didn't mean to hurt you. I was just trying to joke around, but I see now that it wasn't funny."
Child B: "Thank you for saying sorry. I don't like it when people make fun of me like that."
Child A: "I won't do that again. I'll be more careful with my words."

Kindness is essential in communication (Culver, 2024). Even jokes can hurt.

Apologising sincerely and acknowledging the hurt caused helps rebuild trust and maintain friendships.

Not sharing

Unfriendly behaviour:

Child A has a toy that **Child B** wants to play with, but **Child A** refuses to share, saying, "It's mine, you can't play with it."
Child B: "Can I play with that toy? It looks fun!"
Child A: "No, it's mine. You can't play with it."
Child B: "But we're friends. Don't you want to share?"
Child A: "I don't feel like sharing right now."

Friendly communication solution:

Child B: "I understand if you want to play with it right now, but I'd love a turn later."
Child A: "Okay, I can share for a little while. You can have a turn after me."
Child B: "Thanks! I'll wait for my turn."

Sharing and turn-taking build strong friendships (Kennedy-Moore & Mclaughlin, 2017).

Self-leadership: What if I like how I communicate, but everyone else thinks I need to be friendlier? (Self-Awareness, Empathy and Perspective Taking, Communication Skills)

Communication styles are unique. Tone, body language, vocabulary, facial expressions, pace, and skills are on a broad spectrum, influenced by many factors, including personality, temperament, genetics, environment, modelling, character, and values that, when combined, make each person differ significantly. Authenticity is crucial for happiness and well-being, and the goal here is not to make a person change who they are. What decades of experience with tens of thousands of young people have taught me is that everyone seeks connection, and kind, friendly communication skills help create psychological safety for connecting with and including others. The goal is to make things easier for those who struggle, to teach them what they want to learn, and to create an inclusive and compassionate society where diversity is understood and appreciated.

Communication essentials give people a better chance of connection, stemming from our human need to feel safe with others. Our central nervous systems are the first responders when we arrive at a social space. Our survival brain is easily triggered by other people's character and tone if it feels threatening or unkind. I've seen many of my well-intentioned and kind-hearted clients unintentionally speak in a way that feels threatening, and I've helped them soften their tone and use friendlier words. This is much more than a personality clash; it is about a communication style that is universally perceived as threatening, even though it is unintended. Some sound angry when, in reality, their tone reflects that they care deeply about something and are thinking extra hard while communicating, yet it comes across as gruff and abrupt.

Conveying this to a person is never easy because feedback on our social skills feels very personal, especially if we don't yet have the self-awareness to fully understand it or see why it's important. Some people might argue that it's best to leave it alone and let the person be, while others need to adapt and understand the person's verbal and non-verbal communication. While I wholeheartedly believe in compassion, inclusion, and adapting to each other's unique communication and personality styles, I can't ignore the years of suffering for so many of my clients, when, by no fault of their own, guidance wasn't provided, and they truly wish it had been.

Some personalities just find it very difficult to stick to a goal, and Gretchen Rubin's research on expectations helps clarify how personality traits can affect our openness to learning, as well as our friendship and communication skills (Rubin, 2024). Some people decide to improve something, try for a while, and then give up. Others might not see the point in improving, but encouragement from others will give them the motivation to keep going and make progress. Then there are people who need to feel they came up with the idea to improve, to give it a go, and finally, there's the ideal, where someone is driven by internal and external motivation and just gets things done!

The pattern of responding to expectations (what others or we ourselves think we *should* do) is phenomenally diverse. Gretchen Rubin (2017) has identified four main personality tendencies in her research that shape how we learn, behave, and relate to others.

Put simply, for our students, let's imagine friendship learning as a garden where every child is a unique seed, and each needs a little something different to grow kindness, compassion, and respect. Just as every flower grows differently in a garden, each child's personality shapes how they learn the art of friendship. When we can understand and nurture these differences, kindness and compassion don't just get taught; they flourish (Rubin, 2017).

Rubin's four personality tendencies

1. *Upholders like to follow the rules and do what's expected of them. They love ticking off their "to-do" lists and take pride in doing the right thing.*

   How this affects friendship learning: Upholders usually try hard to be kind and fair because they like doing what's right. Sometimes they feel stressed when they think they've broken a "friendship rule."

How can we help support their social-emotional well-being and friendship skill development?

Praise their consistency and kindness (outer expectation).

Encourage flexibility and self-compassion when friendships become challenging (due to inner expectations).

Remind them that making mistakes in friendships is part of learning.

2. *Questioners: Questioners ask why before they do something. They need things to make sense before they join in.*

How this affects friendship learning: Questioners might not follow kindness rules just because "a teacher said so." They'll want to know why kindness matters. Once they understand the reason, they can be loyal and fair friends.

How can we help support their social-emotional well-being and friendship skill development?

Explain the why behind friendship lessons (e.g., "We use kind words because they help others feel safe and happy").

Involve them in problem-solving ("What do you think makes someone a good friend?").

Celebrate their curiosity, which helps them develop a deep understanding of empathy (Rubin, 2017; Ryan & Deci, 2000) (Table 5.1).

Table 5.1 Rubin's four personality tendencies

	Tendency	Seeks	We can help by
Upholder	Clarity and structure.	Learn it's okay to make mistakes.	Encouraging flexibility and self-kindness.
Questioner	Logic and reason.	Understand *why* kindness matters.	Use inquiry-based learning.
Obliger	Connection and support.	Balance helping others and self-care.	Build accountability and boundaries.
Rebel.	Freedom and choice.	Choosing kindness as self-expression.	Offer autonomy and identity-based framing.

3. *Obligers: Obligers love helping others, but sometimes forget to help themselves. They do their best when someone is cheering them on.*
   How this affects friendship learning: They're often kind and helpful friends, but might say "yes" too much, even when they need a break. They can struggle to set boundaries or stand up for themselves.
   How can we help support their social-emotional well-being and friendship skills?
   Give them gentle accountability (e.g., "Let's check in tomorrow about how you handled that friendship problem").
   Praise their empathy and teach healthy boundaries ("You can be kind and say no").
   Utilise team activities that foster mutual support rather than one-sided support (Neff, 2011; Rubin, 2017).
4. *Rebels: Rebels don't like being told what to do, not even by themselves. Rebels love freedom and want to do things their own way.*
   How this affects friendship learning: They might push back against friendship "rules," but they can also be brave, creative friends who stand up for others when they choose to.
   How can we help support their social-emotional well-being and friendship skills?
   Use freedom-based choices ("You can show kindness in your own way. What do you choose?").
   Focus on identity: "You're the kind of person who includes others."
   Frame kindness as self-expression, not obedience (Deci & Ryan, 1985; Rubin 2017).

Role plays

Explain the tendencies to your students, take a look at the adult quiz here for yourself to understand your tendencies and connect these with your students:

https://gretchenrubin.com/quiz/the-four-tendencies-quiz/

Share how helpful it can be to upskill in communicating with different personality types and communication styles.

Provide the following role-play scenarios, and given the significant learning that will occur through these scripts, consider recording the finished product and sharing it at a whole-school assembly and with families in your school community.

The group project puzzle

Characters:

Upholder: Wants to follow the teacher's directions exactly.
Questioner: Keeps asking *why* they have to do it that way.

Clash: The upholder gets frustrated that the questioner won't just get started.
Friendship fix: The questioner explains they work best when they understand *why*, and the upholder agrees to share the teacher's reasoning. They both learn it's okay to ask questions and still stay on track.

A script for this friendship challenge might sound something like this:

Characters: Upholder, Questioner
Scene: Working on a poster for school.
Upholder: Okay, the teacher said to use blue paper and write five facts. Let's start!
Questioner: But why blue paper? Wouldn't yellow look brighter?
Upholder: Because that's what the instructions say!
Questioner: But what's the reason for that rule?
Upholder (sighs): I don't know… maybe so they all match?
Questioner: That makes sense! Okay, blue it is.
Upholder (smiling): Thanks for checking. I like how you think things through!

Lesson: Questioners need reasons; Upholders like structure. Both can respect each other's style.

The playground promise

Characters:

Obliger: Promised to play soccer because friends wanted them to.
Rebel: Doesn't want to follow any plan and keeps changing the game.

Clash: The obliger feels pressured to keep everyone happy, and the rebel feels trapped.

Friendship fix: They decide to take turns—one round of soccer, one round of freestyle play. They both feel respected.

A script for this friendship challenge might sound something like this:

Characters: Obliger, Rebel
Scene: Deciding what to play.
Obliger: Everyone wants to play soccer. Let's do that!
Rebel: Nah, I don't feel like soccer today. Let's make up a new game!
Obliger: But I promised the others…
Rebel: Ugh, promises make it less fun.
Obliger: What if we play one round of soccer, then your new game?
Rebel (grinning): Deal! I'll invent something awesome.

Lesson: Compromise helps when one person needs freedom, and another wants to please others.

The homework hangout

Characters:

Upholder: Wants to finish homework before playing.
Rebel: Says, "I'll do it when I feel like it."

Clash: The upholder feels stressed; the rebel feels bossed around.
Friendship fix: They agree to a short play break first, then both start homework when the rebel *chooses* to. The upholder sees that choice can still lead to responsibility.

A script for this friendship challenge might sound something like this:

Characters: Upholder, Rebel
Scene: After school.
Upholder: Let's do our homework first, then we can play.
Rebel: I'll do it later when I feel like it.
Upholder: But the teacher said it's due tomorrow!
Rebel: I don't like being told when to do things.
Upholder: What if we race—whichever player finishes first chooses the game?
Rebel: Ha! You're on!

Lesson: Offering choice and fun motivates rebels without making them feel controlled.

The science experiment debate

Characters:

Questioner: Wants to test a new way to do the experiment.
Obliger: Wants to follow the teacher's instructions exactly.

Clash: The obliger worries about getting in trouble; the questioner worries they'll miss out on discovering something cool.
Friendship fix: They agree to do it the teacher's way first, then try the new way after for fun, combining safety and curiosity.

A script for this friendship challenge might sound something like this:

Characters: Questioner, Obliger
Scene: In class, doing an experiment.
Questioner: What if we mix the colours in a different order?
Obliger: We can't! The teacher said not to.
Questioner: But maybe it'll look cooler!
Obliger: I don't want to get in trouble.
Questioner: Okay, let's do it her way first, then try mine after.
Obliger: Perfect! We'll learn both ways.

Lesson: Safety and curiosity can work together.

The birthday party plan

Characters:

Rebel: Doesn't want to plan anything in advance.
Upholder: Has already made a detailed party checklist.

Clash: The rebel says, "Let's just see what happens," while the upholder wants everything perfect.
Friendship fix: The upholder plans a few essentials, and the rebel chooses one surprise activity to add, allowing structure and spontaneity to meet.

A script for this friendship challenge might sound something like this:

Characters: Upholder, Rebel
Scene: Planning a party.
Upholder: I made a list: decorations, games, and cake times.

Rebel: Lists? Boring! Let's just see what happens!
Upholder: But what if we forget something?
Rebel: Then we make it up as we go!
Upholder: Hmm… how about I plan the cake, and you plan a surprise game?
Rebel (smiling): Now that's fun!

Lesson: Planning and spontaneity can mix when both sides get a say.

The friendship club rules

Characters:

Upholder: Wants clear club rules.
Obliger: Agrees to all of them, even ones they don't like.
Rebel: Refuses to follow rules.
Questioner: Keeps asking what the rules are for.

Clash: Chaos. Everyone has a different idea of what constitutes fairness.
Friendship fix: They create *shared values* (kindness, respect) instead of strict rules, and everyone feels included and understood.

A script for this friendship challenge might sound something like this:

Characters: Upholder, Obliger, Rebel, Questioner
Scene: Forming a new friendship club.
Upholder: Rule one, we meet every Tuesday.
Rebel: Rules, rules, rules! Yuck.
Obliger: I'll do whatever everyone wants.
Questioner: Why Tuesday? Why not Wednesday?
Upholder (thinking): Okay, maybe instead of strict rules, we make values, like kindness and respect.
Rebel: I like that!
Questioner: That's a good reason.
Obliger: I'm in!

Lesson: Shared values work better than strict rules for different personalities.

The cleaning crew

Characters:

Obliger: Cleans up even when others don't.
Questioner: Says, "Why clean up if it's just going to get messy again?"

Upholder: Reminds everyone it's the rule.
Rebel: Says, "You can't make me!"

Clash: The room stays messy, and feelings get hurt.
Friendship fix: They turn it into a *clean-up race,* and everyone works together in their own way. The rebel likes the challenge; the obliger feels supported.

A script for this friendship challenge might sound something like this:

Characters: Upholder, Obliger, Questioner, Rebel.
Scene: Cleaning up after an art lesson.
Upholder: Time to clean up, everyone.
Obliger: I'll do it all!
Rebel: You can't make me.
Questioner: Why clean up if we'll paint again tomorrow?
Upholder: Because it's respectful to share a clean space.
Questioner: Okay, that's fair.
Rebel: What if we turn it into a race? Fastest team wins!
Obliger: Great idea! Ready, set, go!

Lesson: When everyone's needs are heard, teamwork feels fun and fair.

The talent show trouble

Characters:

Upholder: Practices every day to be ready.
Rebel: Performs each time differently.
Questioner: Keeps suggesting "better" ideas.

Clash: The upholder feels stressed when others change plans.
Friendship fix: They learn that creativity can still shine within structure, and each gets a short act to perform *their* way.

A script for this friendship challenge might sound something like this:

Characters: Upholder, Rebel, Questioner
Scene: Rehearsing for a class talent show.
Upholder: We said we'd do the dance in this order!
Rebel: I changed it. It's much better this way.
Questioner: Why not try both and see which looks better?

Upholder: Hmm… okay, let's compare.
Rebel: Fine, but my version's better.
(They perform both versions and laugh.)
Upholder: I like how different we all are!

Lesson: Differences can make creative teamwork shine.

The group game glitch.

Characters:

Obliger: Goes along with everyone's ideas.
Questioner: Asks too many "why" questions mid-game.
Rebel: Ignores the rules.
Upholder: Keeps correcting everyone.

Clash: The fun fades fast.
Friendship fix: They pause to laugh about how differently they play, then agree on one simple goal: *have fun, not win* and cooperation returns.

A script for this friendship challenge might sound something like this:

Characters: Upholder, Obliger, Rebel, Questioner
Scene: Playing a board game.
Upholder: You must roll the dice before moving.
Rebel: I'll move first, it's faster.
Questioner: Why is that even a rule?
Obliger: I'll just do whatever makes everyone happy.
(They all start talking at once.)
Upholder: Wait! Let's make one rule: have fun, not fight.
Rebel: I like that one.
Questioner: Makes sense.
Obliger: Me too!

Lesson: Relationships matter more than being right.

The art project argument

Characters:

Questioner: Wants to explore a creative twist.
Obliger: Worries the teacher won't like it.

Rebel: Paints something wild and different.
Upholder: Sticks strictly to the example.

Clash: Everyone thinks the others are "doing it wrong."
Friendship fix: The teacher reminds them that art is about *expression, not perfection*. They realise different styles make the mural beautiful.

A script for this friendship challenge might sound something like this:

Characters: Upholder, Questioner, Rebel, Obliger
Scene: Making a mural together.
Upholder: The example shows we should use blue for the sky.
Rebel: I'm painting it green!
Questioner: But why blue anyway?
Obliger: The teacher said to, so I will.
(They all stop and look at the mural.)
Upholder: Wait. Your green sky looks amazing.
Rebel (smiling): Told you!
Questioner: Maybe the rule is just to *be creative*.
Obliger: Then we're all doing it right!

Lesson: Everyone's approach can add beauty and value.

> **Reflection questions for students after each role play**
> How did each character's personality tendency affect communication?
> What helped them understand each other better?
> How can we show kindness and flexibility when someone thinks or
>   acts differently from us?
>
> **Whole class reflection:** After completing the role plays, invite students to share:
>
> Which personality style feels most like you?
> What personality style feels easy or hard for you to get along with,
>   and why?
> What's one thing you can do to show kindness to someone who has
>   a different tendency from you?

When to forgive, when to hold on. (Conflict Resolution and Problem Solving, Empathy and Perspective Taking, Self-Awareness)

As Nelson Mandela once said,

> Resentment is like drinking poison and then hoping it will kill your enemies.

Harbouring every conflict between friends can upset the balance of accepting and understanding each other's levels of awareness and development. It's important to lead by example as adults, as some children, often those who are neurodivergent or have experienced traumatic childhoods, can struggle with emotional regulation and social behaviour, unintentionally upsetting other children through repetitive behaviour. You will notice reference is made in this lesson to "less forgivable" rather than "unforgivable" to keep children open-minded and to account for student diversity.

Dr Eileen Kennedy-Moore, Psychologist and friendship expert, teaches us that holding on to grudges is emotionally costly. Far too often, young people get caught up in mistakes made by other children and avoid reparation and moving forward. While some friendships are not worth holding onto because of intentional cruelty and repetitive conflict, often in childhood, things can be moved forward from. Learning this early on in life will help with adult relationships later, when the stakes are often much higher.

Dr Kennedy-Moore offers the following advice for children to determine whether forgiveness is a path to follow in a friendship in trouble (Kennedy-Moore & McLaughlin, 2017).

If it only happened one time, and it probably won't happen again, let it go.
If your friend didn't do it on purpose, let it go.
If it wasn't that bad, let it go.
If your friend is sorry, let it go.
If it was just a mistake, and the friend is usually kind, let it go.
If it happened more than a month ago, let it go.

> Holding onto resentment is emotionally costly. Sometimes, forgiveness is the right thing to do, not because the other person deserves it, but because we deserve not to be weighed down with bitterness.
>
> (Kennedy-Moore, 2025)

Project this forgiveness framework on the board and help your students develop their awareness and understanding of it.

Forgiveness role plays

Provide students with the following scenarios and ask them to work towards a solution in which forgiveness is possible and help from an adult might be needed, to nip a conflict in the bud and work toward a friendly resolution, followed by forgiveness. Remind them to refer back to the forgiveness model by Dr Kennedy-Moore.

Role plays for younger students

Taking a toy without asking

Scenario: Alex grabs Jamie's toy car without asking.
Forgivable outcome: Alex apologises and returns it. Jamie forgives, and they
   play together.
A less forgivable outcome: Alex takes the toy, intentionally breaks it, and
   refuses to apologise.

Interrupting during a game

Scenario: Mia keeps interrupting Noah during a game of board.
Forgivable outcome: Mia realises she is interrupting, says sorry, and waits
   her turn.
Less forgivable outcome: Mia keeps interrupting and snatches the game
   pieces when Noah tries to explain.

Spreading a rumour

Scenario: Sam tells a story about Lily that isn't completely true.
Forgivable outcome: Sam admits to the mistake and apologises; Lily accepts
   and moves on.
Less forgivable outcome: Sam continues to spread false stories to discredit
   Lily.

Accidental bumping

Scenario: Ethan accidentally bumps into Sara and knocks her water bottle over.

Forgivable outcome: Ethan apologises and helps with the cleanup. Sara forgives him.

Less forgivable outcome: Ethan bumps her on purpose and laughs when her drink spills.

Not sharing materials

Scenario: Zoe refuses to share the coloured pencils during art time.

Forgivable outcome: Zoe decides to share after being reminded, and the group works happily.

Less forgivable outcome: Zoe refuses to share even after repeated reminders and snatches pencils from others.

Calling names

Scenario: Liam calls Riley a mean nickname.

Forgivable outcome: Liam apologises and promises not to say it again. Riley accepts the apology.

Less forgivable outcome: Liam keeps calling Riley names to upset them on purpose.

Excluding someone

Scenario: Ava doesn't invite Jack to play during recess.

Forgivable outcome: Ava realises her mistake, invites Jack, and they all play together.

Less forgivable outcome: Ava keeps excluding Jack every time and encourages others not to play with him.

Taking credit for work

Scenario: Max presents a drawing Jack made as his own.

Forgivable outcome: Max admits it was Jack's work and gives him credit.

Less forgivable outcome: Max insists it's his work and refuses to acknowledge Jack's contribution.

Accidental hitting

Scenario: Sophia accidentally hits Emma with a ball during PE.

Forgivable outcome: Sophia apologises, helps Emma, and Emma forgives her.

Less forgivable outcome: Sophia throws the ball at Emma on purpose repeatedly.

Breaking a promise

Scenario: Oliver promises to help Mia with a class task, but forgets.

Forgivable outcome: Oliver apologises and makes it up by helping next time.

Less forgivable outcome: Oliver lies and says he helped when he didn't, and refuses to help at all.

Forgiveness role plays for older students

Cheating in a group project

Scenario: Jordan copies parts of Taylor's work without asking.

Forgivable outcome: Jordan admits the mistake, apologises, and rewrites the work properly.

Less forgivable outcome: Jordan continues to take credit for Taylor's work and refuses to acknowledge their contribution.

Spreading a hurtful post online

Scenario: Mia shares a picture of Ethan online with a mean caption.

Forgivable outcome: Mia realises it was hurtful, deletes the post, and apologises.

Less forgivable outcome: Mia continues to post mean content about Ethan and encourages others to comment.

Breaking a confidence

Scenario: Liam tells a secret that Olivia shared with him.

Forgivable outcome: Liam apologises and promises not to tell anyone else. Olivia forgives him.

Less forgivable outcome: Liam deliberately shares more secrets to embarrass Olivia.

Arguing over team roles

Scenario: Ava refuses to take on the assigned role in a sports team.

Forgivable outcome: Ava accepts the role after discussion and participates respectfully.

Less forgivable outcome: Ava refuses, deliberately disrupts the team, and insults teammates.

Excluding someone from a study group

Scenario: Noah doesn't include Sara in a study group for an important assignment.

Forgivable outcome: Noah apologises and invites Sara to join them, and they work together.

Less forgivable outcome: Noah purposely excludes Sara again and tells others not to include her either.

Mocking someone's opinion

Scenario: Max laughs at Zoe's idea during a class debate.

Forgivable outcome: Max apologises and listens to Zoe's perspective.

Less forgivable outcome: Max continues mocking Zoe and tries to turn others against her.

Using someone's belongings without permission

Scenario: Sophia uses Emma's laptop without asking.

Forgivable outcome: Sophia apologises, returns it, and asks for permission before borrowing next time.

A less forgivable outcome: Sophia continues to use Emma's laptop, changes settings, or deletes files.

Interrupting or talking over someone

Scenario: Oliver frequently interrupts during class discussions.

Forgivable outcome: Oliver realises he is interrupting, apologises, and waits for his turn.

Less forgivable outcome: Oliver ignores requests to stop and continues to disrupt others.

Rumour about a teacher

Scenario: Ethan spreads a rumour about a teacher online.

Forgivable outcome: Ethan deletes the rumour and apologises, realising it was inappropriate.

Less forgivable outcome: Ethan continues spreading lies to make others dislike the teacher.

Stealing someone's achievement

Scenario: Mia claims she got the top score in a test, even though it was Noah.
Forgivable outcome: Mia admits the truth and congratulates Noah.
Less forgivable outcome: Mia insists it's hers, brags about it, and tries to discredit Noah.

Forgiveness reflection

Bring your group together to share a time you were forgiven for something you did and later regretted. Next, present your students with the following role plays to practice ways to show forgiveness and to keep them thinking about the difference between forgivable and less forgivable challenges.

Group work disagreement

Forgivable: Ella interrupted James in group work. James thought, *"She's just excited."* He forgave her by saying, "Let's both share our ideas and then vote."
Harder: Ella dismissed James' idea, saying, *"Yours are never good."* This was intentional, making forgiveness very difficult.

Being left out of a game

Forgivable: Luca didn't ask Harry to join the basketball team. Harry thought, *"He probably didn't notice me."* He asked for forgiveness by saying, "Can I join the next round?" and Luca said, "Yes."
Harder: Luca said, *"You can't play, you're not good."* This was a direct rejection, so forgiving was harder.

Sharing secrets

Forgivable: Amira told others something Sienna shared, not realising it was private. Sienna thought, *"She didn't know it was a secret."* She forgave by saying, "Next time, can you check before telling?"
Harder: Amira spread Sienna's secret on purpose to the class. Forgiveness was much harder because trust was broken.

Jealousy in competition

Forgivable: Ben rolled his eyes when Ava won a contest. Ava thought, *"He's just upset with himself."* She forgave him by smiling and not taking it personally.

Harder: Ben told others, *"Ava only won because she got easy words."* This was meant to hurt her, so forgiving was harder.

Accidentally ignoring someone

Forgivable: Zara didn't wave back when Mia said hi in the yard. Mia thought, *"Maybe she didn't see me."* She forgave her by greeting her again later.

Harder: Zara looked at Mia and whispered to another friend, *"Don't talk to her."* This was a purposeful exclusion, making forgiveness difficult.

Joking that goes too far

Forgivable: Tom teased Alex about being slow at running, then quickly said, *"I'm just joking!"* Alex forgave him by replying, "Okay, but can you joke about something else?"

Harder: Tom kept calling Alex "slowpoke" in front of everyone. Forgiveness was harder because it turned into repeated teasing.

Borrowing without asking

Forgivable: Chloe borrowed Maya's coloured pencils without asking. Maya thought, *"Maybe she forgot to ask."* She forgave her by saying, "Next time, can you check with me first?"

Harder: Chloe hid Maya's pencils on purpose and laughed when Maya couldn't find them. That felt mean, so forgiving was harder.

Not keeping a promise

Forgivable: Ryan promised to sit with Jack at lunch, but forgot and sat somewhere else. Jack thought, *"Maybe he got distracted."* He forgave by asking Ryan to sit together the next day.

Harder: Ryan told Jack, *"I never wanted to sit with you anyway."* That was deliberately hurtful, making forgiveness very hard.

Taking credit

Forgivable: During art class, Lily showed the teacher her drawing and forgot to mention that Sofia helped. Sofia thought, *"She probably didn't mean to leave me out."* She forgave her by saying, "Let's both show it next time."

Harder: Lily told the teacher, *"I did all the work; Sofia didn't help at all."* That was dishonest and unfair, so forgiving was harder.

Rumours

Forgivable: Josh told a story he thought was funny, but didn't realise it embarrassed Ethan. Ethan thought, *"He probably didn't know it would upset me."* He forgave him by saying, "Please don't tell that story again."

Harder: Josh made up a rumour about Ethan to get others laughing. Forgiveness was much harder because it was intentional.

How enthusiastic and warm communication skills can help with forgiveness

Different personalities, cultures, genetic expression, and neurobiological hardwiring all affect a person's social communication styles. Being greeted with enthusiasm and warmth is something cultures around the world agree is received with appreciation, while ignoring, excluding, and communicating harshly is not (Liu, 2018). Teaching young people the art of showing warmth and happiness towards others can strengthen bonds, increase psychological safety, and release dopamine, serotonin, and oxytocin, while opening more social doors than leaving this skill out of the equation (Culver, 2024). Genuine warmth and enthusiasm are skills that aren't as easy to develop as they come from a place of emotion, and they are very hard to "act out." The best way for a child to do this is to encourage adults in the child's environment to display warmth and enthusiasm. The more children see adults showing warmth and enthusiasm towards each other, and even better, experience adults showing warmth and enthusiasm towards them, the more likely this will come naturally to them. When a person is warm and enthusiastic towards others.

Neurodivergence and friendly communication. (Self-Awareness, Empathy and Perspective Taking, Communication Skills)

We've covered many ways children can communicate pro-socially. It's important to remember that not everyone will find this easy or align with its values. In my experience, my clients have always been grateful for the opportunity to learn more about these techniques, which help them feel more comfortable and confident socially. Helping a child understand that their verbal and non-verbal communication can be confusing to others in a neuroaffirming way involves providing them with supportive, empathetic, and non-punitive strategies. The goal is to help all children develop awareness and empathy, without shaming or stigmatising them. Here are some strategies to approach this:

1. Create a safe and non-judgmental space for discussion

Why: Children may not fully understand the impact of their behaviour on others, especially if they have a communication difference. Creating a supportive environment where they feel safe to discuss their actions is crucial.

How: Use gentle, neutral language. Avoid labelling their behaviour as "bad" or "wrong." Instead, frame the conversation in terms of understanding and improving how they connect with others.

Example: "I noticed that when you spoke to your friend, they seemed upset. Can we talk about what happened?"

2. Use visual and concrete examples

Why: Children, especially those who are neurodivergent, often benefit from visual aids or concrete examples to understand abstract concepts like emotional impact or body language.

How: Use role-play, social stories, or video clips to demonstrate how certain words or body language affect others. Show the child what "hurtful" or confusing communication looks like and contrast it with other methods of communication.

Example: Show a video of two children talking, then pause to discuss how the other child's crossed arms and harsh tone might make the first feel.

3. Focus on identifying and labelling emotions

Why: Helping a child recognise and name their own emotions, as well as the emotions of others, enables them to understand the social context of their words and actions.

How: Use emotion charts, pictures, or apps that help children learn about facial expressions and body language related to emotions. Discuss how different emotions (e.g., frustration, sadness, excitement) might be communicated through words or body language.

Example: "When you're upset, you might say things in a louder voice, or your face might look angry. Let's try to notice how other people might feel when they hear that."

4. Use positive reinforcement for friendly communication

Why: Positive reinforcement encourages the child to practice more pro-social communication by acknowledging and rewarding their efforts in a supportive way.

How: When a child uses kind or considerate communication, offer praise and recognition. Reinforce the connection between their words and the positive outcomes for themselves and others.

Example: "I noticed you spoke to your friend really gently. That made them smile. You're such a kind person, and it warms my heart to see it come out in your words."

5. Model neuroaffirming communication

Why: Children learn by example. Kindness and bullying are all learnt behaviours. Modelling how kind and respectful communication, including non-verbal cues, is a great way to show all students that kindness and inclusion are the only acceptable ways to behave in your school. Neurodivergence is celebrated, valued, and appreciated always.

6. Break down social expectations into manageable steps

Why: Children may have difficulty understanding or applying social rules, especially if they're neurodivergent. Breaking complex social expectations into smaller, concrete steps can make them more achievable, giving them equal access to social knowledge that may come more easily to their peers.

7. Teach self-regulation strategies

Why: Sometimes, children are unaware of how their words or actions affect others because they are struggling with emotional regulation or impulsivity.

How: Teach the child self-regulation techniques such as deep breathing, counting to 10, or taking a short break before responding in situations that might trigger a strong emotional reaction.

Example: "When you're feeling frustrated, you can stop and take three deep breaths before you speak. That way, you can choose your words carefully."

8. Use social scripts and role-playing

Why: Children with neurodivergent traits often benefit from structured approaches to social interaction. Social scripts offer a clear, repeatable model for communicating effectively in various situations.

How: Provide scripts for common social situations, like asking to join a game or apologising for a mistake. Use role-playing to practice these scripts in a supportive environment.

Example: "If you accidentally hurt someone's feelings, you can say, 'I'm sorry I made you feel bad. I didn't mean to.' Let's practice this together."

9. Be patient and avoid punitive responses

Why: Shaming or punishing a child for their communication style will increase anxiety and social withdrawal. It's also unfair and unkind. We can help children grow through guidance, mutual respect, and understanding, along with regular communication about their own goals and needs, not just the skills adults think they should develop.

How: When addressing hurtful communication, approach the child with compassion, kindness, and patience. Always recognise that they may not fully understand the impact of their behaviour. Focus on teaching and guiding them toward better choices rather than punitive measures.

Example: Instead of saying "That was rude," try saying, "I understand you were upset, but that comment might have hurt your friend's feelings. Let's talk about what could be said instead."

By using these strategies, children can develop a greater awareness of how their words and body language land, learn to regulate their emotions, and improve their communication in a supportive and encouraging way.

This approach fosters empathy and helps them build meaningful, positive relationships. Teaching these skills provides neurodivergent children with an opportunity to access knowledge and skills that come easily to many of their peers. Whether they choose to use them or feel comfortable using them is up to them, but not sharing this social knowledge with them can also make their lives much harder.

Key takeaways from Chapter 5

Friendly communication forms the foundation of strong, healthy friendships, with both verbal and nonverbal skills playing crucial roles (CASEL, 2023; Goleman, 1995; Kennedy-Moore & Mclaughlin, 2017).

- Self-awareness, empathy, and respectful listening are essential for building trust and understanding in peer interactions (Neff, 2011; Ryan & Deci, 2000; UNESCO, 2022).
- Students can learn the impact of their words, recognise and respond to non-verbal cues, and appreciate the diversity of communication styles, including those related to neurodivergence (CASEL, 2023; UNESCO, 2022).
- Emphasising inclusion, mutual respect, and forgiveness fosters resilience and supports social-emotional wellbeing (CASEL, 2023; UNESCO, 2022).

Call to action

Practice friendly communication every day! Try a new "green-light" word, give a genuine compliment, or be a "listening detective" with a friend or family member. Celebrate your unique style and help others feel welcome— because every classroom is better when everyone shines!

References

CASEL. (2023). What is SEL? Collaborative for academic, social, and emotional learning. https://casel.org/fundamentals-of-sel/

Culver, C. S. (2024, November 14). *The science of kindness: How acts of kindness transform the classroom.* Orange Sparrow. https://www.orangesparrow.org/the-kind-voice/the-science-of-kindness

Deci, E. L., & Ryan, R. M. (1985). *Intrinsic motivation and self-determination in human behavior* (1st ed.). Springer US. https://doi.org/10.1007/978-1-4899-2271-7

Goleman, D. (1995). *Emotional intelligence: Why it can matter more than IQ.* Bantam Books.

Kennedy-Moore, E. (2025). *Open door for parents | Webinars.* Open Door for Parents. https://learn.eileenkennedymoore.com/

Kennedy-Moore, E., & Mclaughlin, C. (2017). *Growing friendships: A kid's guide to making and keeping friends.* Beyond Words.

Liu, L. (2018). Reconsidering intercultural communication competence development in different social patterns - Starting from the study of greetings. *International Journal for Cross-Disciplinary Subjects in Education, 9*(2), 3393–3399. https://doi.org/10.20533/ijcdse.2042.6364.2018.0454

Neff, K. D. (2011). Self-compassion, self-esteem, and well-being. *Social and Personality Psychology Compass, 5*(1), 1–12. https://doi.org/10.1111/j.1751-9004.2010.00330.x

Rubin, G. (2014). *Are you an Upholder, a Questioner, a Rebel, or an Obliger?* Retrieved from https://gretchenrubin.com/articles/are-you-an-upholder-a-questioner-a-rebel-or-an-obliger

Rubin, G. (2024). *Getting Started: The Four Tendencies.* Gretchen Rubin. https://gretchenrubin.com/four-tendencies/

Rubin, G. (2017). *The four tendencies: The indispensable personality profiles that reveal how to make your life better (and other people's lives better, too).* https://www.barnesandnoble.com/w/the-four-tendencies-gretchen-rubin/1126242312

Ryan, R. M., & Deci, E. L. (2000). Self-determination theory and the facilitation of intrinsic motivation, social development, and wellbeing. *American Psychologist, 55*(1), 68–78. https://doi.org/10.1037/0003-066X.55.1.68

UNESCO. (2022). *Social and emotional learning: Policy and practice.* United Nations Educational, Scientific and Cultural Organization. https://en.unesco.org/themes/sel

Appendix: Friendship toolkit and fun extras!

Friendship fun challenge ideas (for teachers and students)

Create your own "Green-Light Words" poster for the classroom.

Keep a "Kindness Journal" and record one kind thing you say or do each day.

Make up a class handshake or greeting that everyone can learn.

Hold a "Listening Detective" badge ceremony for students who demonstrate excellent listening skills.

Set a weekly 'Friendship Quest'—like including someone new at lunch or recess.

Kindness, compassion, and inclusion

> Kindness is much more than a simple act; it's a gentle offering of psychological safety and warmth, allowing connection to fall gently into place.

The kindness adventure quest. (Empathy and Perspective Taking, Communication Skills, Self-Awareness, Conflict Resolution, and Problem Solving)

Get ready, explorers! This chapter is your invitation to a grand adventure where every act of kindness, every spark of compassion, and every moment of inclusion help build a school where everyone belongs. You'll collect "kindness gems" along the way and discover how your words and actions can change your school for the better!

Small gestures transform classrooms, families, and playgrounds. In this chapter, students will discover how kindness, compassion, and inclusion create belonging and strengthen friendships (Hosoda & Estrada, 2024). They'll explore how personal biases shape relationships and learn that neurodivergence offers unique strengths (White et al., 2023). Through discussion and reflection, students will practice fairness and gain insight into the impact of their actions, understanding that inclusivity benefits everyone (Bear, 2020).

DOI: 10.4324/9781003617570-6

Setting the scene (Chapter overview)

Kindness, compassion, and inclusion are never wasted—they build lasting hope and connection (Hosoda & Estrada, 2024). Decades of research show these values support both individuals and communities, enhancing psychological safety and well-being (Bear, 2020; Jennings & Greenberg, 2009).

Those hardest to include often need kindness most. Teaching self-leadership and self-regulation helps everyone and shifts school culture toward inclusion (Hamre & Pianta, 2001).

Kindness and inclusion help everyone feel valued and foster authenticity. Inclusive schools embrace diversity so every student belongs (White et al., 2023).

Spotting the skills in action (Observation and Reflection) (Self-Awareness, Empathy, and Perspective Taking)

Lucy's first mural

At Castlewood Primary, art class was everyone's favourite, except for Lucy. She loved art but struggled in class. Paintbrushes never worked as she wanted, and her pictures looked "different." Loud chatter and bright lights made lessons overwhelming, so Lucy often sat by the window, thinking of her family and her dog Juno.

Lucy was autistic. Her teacher, Ms Hallop, understood how Lucy saw the world and worked to make her feel safe and comfortable in class. Her classmates didn't yet understand autism, and Ms Hallop knew this was unhelpful.

One morning, Ms Hallop announced, "Today we're making a mural about kindness and inclusion! You'll work in teams." Teams formed quickly, but Lucy's didn't. She waited, used to being last chosen, feeling embarrassed. Ms Hallop paired her with Ava, Jamal, and Noah. Ava whispered, "She always takes ages." Noah said, "Let's just give her a small part." Ms Hallop reminded them, "Everyone's ideas matter. Sometimes unique minds see what others miss." Still, the group ignored Lucy's quiet suggestions. While they drew smiling faces, Lucy traced a blue swirl. Jamal asked, "What's that?" Lucy replied, "It's kindness. When someone is kind, it feels like calm waves inside me." Jamal said, "I never thought of kindness as a colour." Lucy smiled. "I feel colours. Each emotion has one."

Lucy thought for a long moment. "Golden. Like sunlight that doesn't hurt your eyes."

For the first time, Ava and Jamal leaned in, their interest piqued. "That's beautiful," Ava whispered. Ms Hallop smiled from across the room, watching the small group begin to glow with curiosity instead of judgment.

Lucy suggested adding colours for feelings: green for peace, red for courage, purple for belonging. Noah said, "But people don't look like that." Ava replied, "It's not weird. It's how Lucy sees the world. Maybe we'd notice more colours too."

By week's end, their team was last to finish, and others teased them. But when Ms Hallop revealed their mural, everyone gasped.

The mural shimmered with swirling colours that blended yet kept their shape—like people in a community. In the centre, open hands held a golden circle, with smaller hands reaching out. Noah whispered, "It looks like the world... but full of feelings." Lucy smiled. "That's what kindness does, it connects our colours."

Ms Hallop said, "You each added your own colour—together, you made something extraordinary." After that, Lucy's classmates listened and respected her needs. When someone new joined, Lucy was the first to say, "You can add your colour too."

At the end-of-year assembly, the mural was unveiled in sunlight, gleaming in the school hall.

Ava whispered, "Kindness is seeing someone's colour, even if it's not what you expected." Lucy nodded. Ms Hallop asked Ava to repeat it to the assembly, then said, "That's compassion, seeing with your heart."

As the crowd clapped, the golden circle seemed to glow. True inclusion isn't about fitting everyone into the same lines, it's about widening the lines so everyone can shine.

Reflection for parents and educators

What did you learn from this story?

What do you think about Lucy's grades in art? Could anything be changed there to show kindness, compassion, and inclusion, making it fair for her?

Can you think of a neurodivergent person in history who made big changes to the world that you can share to inspire children?

What do you think could be done differently to make the world kinder, compassionate, and inclusive?

Reflection for students

What was something new you learnt about neurodivergence from this story?

Ms Hallop was amazing, wasn't she? Is there anything she could have improved on?

Personal bias and friendships

Appreciating others despite differences strengthens communities. Teaching about bias early builds harmony (Zins et al., 2004).

Group brainstorm and discussion about personal bias. (Self-Awareness, Empathy, and perspective taking, Communication skills)

Personal preferences and assumptions influence relationships. Unfair judgments based on differences can block friendships (Bear, 2020).

You can start with a basic definition like: "Bias is when we like or don't like someone, for reasons that aren't fair, like because of what they look like, where they come from, or how they think or speak."

After explaining bias, invite students to discuss and add examples of different kinds of bias using the following categories (Figure 6.1).

SAY NO TO BIAS
EVERYONE BELONGS

APPEARANCE BIAS

Picking friends for how they look (clothes, culture, hair, etc.).

BEHAVIOUR BIAS

Judging or excluding others for how they act or what they like.

STEREOTYPES

Assuming things about someone's home, likes, or gender.

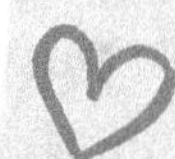

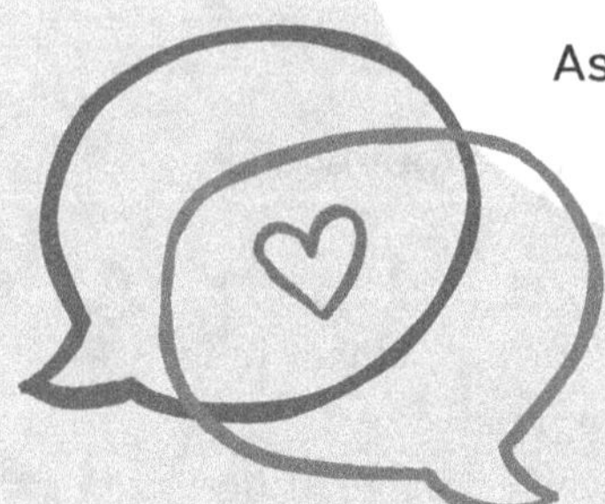

BEING DIFFERENT MAKES OUR SCHOOL STRONGER.

CELEBRATE WHAT MAKES YOU AND OTHERS UNIQUE.

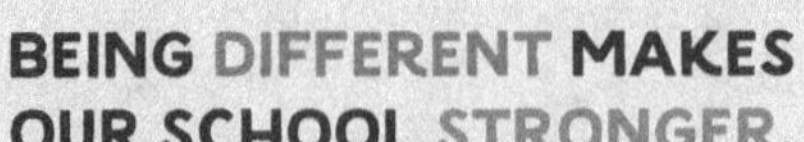

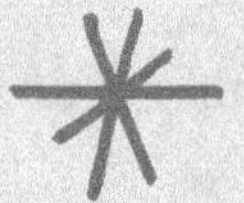

Personal bias mural or poster. (Self-Awareness, Communication skills)

Create a classroom reminder about personal bias for ongoing reference. Consider video clips or set goals to talk to someone new.

Bias role plays. (Empathy and perspective taking, Communication skills, Conflict resolution, and problem solving)

Divide students into groups to explore bias, pairing them with classmates they don't usually work with. Find ways to record or share what they learn.

Accent bias

Scenario: A new student speaks with a strong accent. Some children laugh and mimic their voice.

Teacher prompts:
"Let's try acting out what happens when the class laughs."
"Now, let's try showing kindness instead. What could you say to help the new student feel welcome?"

Debrief questions:
How do you think the new student felt when people laughed at them?
What words or actions helped them feel included?
Have you ever heard someone speak in a different way? How did you respond?

Racial bias

Scenario: A child with darker skin asks to join a group game. Someone says, "You can't play, brown people can't play with us."

Teacher prompts:
"Let's see what it feels like to be told you can't play."
"Now, let's act out how to invite them kindly."

Debrief questions:
How would you feel if someone left you out for how you look?
What's something kind you could say to welcome them?
Why is it important that everyone is included?

Disability bias

Scenario: A student in a wheelchair wants to join a chasing game. Another says, "You can't play, you're too slow."

Teacher prompts:

"First, let's act out what happens when they're left out."
"Now, can we find a way to adapt the game so everyone can join?"

Debrief questions:

How did the student in the wheelchair feel in each version?
What are some creative ways to make games fair for everyone?
Why is it important to change the game instead of leaving someone out?

Learning disability bias

Scenario: A child struggles with reading. A classmate says, "You're dumb, I don't want you in my group."

Teacher prompts:

"Act out the hurtful version first."
"Now, how could the group make sure everyone has a role?"

Debrief questions:

How does it feel to be excluded because of a challenge?
What strengths can we notice in people who learn differently?
How can groups share tasks fairly?

Gender stereotypes

Scenario: A boy wants to play with dolls. Someone says, "That's for girls."

Teacher prompts:

"Let's try acting out the teasing version."
"Now, what would it look like if classmates supported his choice?"

Debrief questions:

How do gender stereotypes stop people from having fun?
Why is it okay for everyone to enjoy all kinds of toys?
Can you think of something you enjoy that others might think is unusual for your gender?

Behavioural bias

Scenario: A child who sometimes struggles with self-control wants to join a group. Someone says, "No, you always mess things up."

Teacher prompts:

"Show us what it looks like to be rejected right away."
"Now, let's practice giving someone a chance while setting kind boundaries."

Debrief questions:

How does it feel to always be judged by past behaviour?
What are fair ways to give someone another chance?
Why is it important to see people for who they are today, not just yesterday?

Socioeconomic bias

Scenario: A child doesn't have the newest sneakers. Another says, "You can't play with us because your shoes are old."

Teacher prompts:

"Let's act out the hurtful version first."
"Now, what could friends say instead to make them feel valued?"

Debrief questions:

How might someone feel being teased for what they own?
Do our belongings make us better or worse friends?
What matters more than clothes or shoes in a friendship?

Religious and cultural bias

Scenario: A child brings different food for lunch. Some laugh and say, "That's gross."

Teacher prompts:

"Let's try teasing first."
"Now, can you act out a curious and respectful way to ask about the food?"

Debrief Questions:

How would it feel to be laughed at for your food?
What could you say to learn more about someone's culture in a kind way?
Why is it good to try new foods or respect different ones?

Stereotyping personalities

Scenario: A quiet child wants to join the talent show. Someone says, "You're too shy to do that."

Teacher prompts:

"Act out the discouraging response."

"Now, show us what it looks like to encourage someone to give it a go."

Debrief questions:

How does it feel when people assume what you can or can't do?

Why is it important to let people choose for themselves?

How can you support a friend who's nervous to try something new?

Friendship bias (exclusion)

Scenario: A child asks to sit at a lunch table. Another says, "No, only our friends can sit here."

Teacher Prompts:

"Let's act out what it feels like to be told you can't sit there."

"Now, let's show what it looks like to invite them in."

Debrief Questions:

How does it feel to be left out of a group?

Why do cliques hurt people's feelings?

What's a simple way to make sure everyone feels welcome at lunch?

Finding common ground instead of fixating on our biases. (Empathy and Perspective Taking, Communication Skills, Self-Awareness)

Friendships start with shared interests. Building genuine connections strengthens a sense of belonging and wellbeing (Zins et al., 2004).

Friendship bingo

Give each student a friendship bingo card to find classmates with shared interests. They can write names or tick boxes as they go (Table 6.1).

Friendship Bingo: Find friends who match the boxes and write their names in!

Table 6.1 Friendship bingo card

Likes the same fruit as you	Has/hasn't got a pet	Watches a TV show you like	Likes to do the same thing you like to do after school	Likes similar music
Finds Maths easy/hard	Prefers quiet/ prefers noise	Is looking forward to something you're looking forward to	Plays/ doesn't play video games	Has been to a place you love
Likes/dislikes watching sport	Likes/dislikes board games	FREE SPACE	Can/can't speak another language	Has/hasn't moved house before
Wants something you want and isn't allowed to have it	Likes animals	Has a similar talent to you	Has/ doesn't have a sibling	Parents were/ weren't born in another country
Has the same birthday month as you	Has the same hobby as you	Likes/doesn't like to be creative	Shares the same favourite teacher as you	Enjoys doing the same thing you do to relax

Pair students with someone new for board or card games. Rotating partners helps everyone practice open-mindedness and courage.

Friendship bias self-reflection. (Self-Awareness, Empathy, and Perspective Taking)

Guide students to reflect privately on meeting someone new and why they liked or didn't like them. No need to share aloud.

The ways bias hurts others and can stop a great friendship from even beginning

Group discussion: When someone judges you on something that's not in your control, like your appearance, background, or interests, it's unfair, unkind, mean-spirited, and can really hurt your feelings.

Ask your students to consider other factors that might bias them. Ask them to hold that in their mind for a moment. Then ask the question:

How would you feel if someone said, "I don't want to be your friend because (insert bias)"?
Can you think of a time when your feelings were hurt because someone decided something about you that's biased, without getting to know you? How did it feel?

Remind your students that it is essential to treat others the way you want to be treated, and that everyone has the right to feel safe and to belong at school.

Personal bias rap. (Communication Skills, Self-Awareness)

Share this rap and invite students to create their own. Consider using it on a themed day.
No way to bias. A call & response rap.

Adult: Yo, what do we say?
Students: No way to bias, not today!
Adult: If someone's different, what's our view?
Students: That makes them awesome, just like you!
Adult: Culture, accent, how we talk,
Students: Everyone belongs when we walk the walk!
Adult: Neurodivergent, shy, or loud,
Students: We're all unique, we all make the crowd!
Adult: When someone's left out, what do we do?
Students: Step in, speak up, and include too!
Adult: What's our rule, clear and true?
Students: Kindness first, in all we do!

ALL TOGETHER (chant).

No way to bias, nah, not today!
We lift each other up in every way.
Different hearts, minds, moves, and tunes,
We all shine bright like stars and moons!

Being a bystander when someone is being mean, is it kind, compassionate or inclusive? (Self-Awareness, Empathy and Perspective Taking, Conflict Resolution and Problem Solving, Communication Skills)

Being accountable for social mistakes is hard. Even kind people can act unkindly when overwhelmed. Standing up to bullying is complicated—sometimes it's not safe or easy, and bystanders can freeze from stress or fear.

Before you begin, remind your class that every day brings new choices to be brave, kind, and true to yourself—even when it's hard. Here's a story that shows how even the smallest decisions can make a huge difference.

Let students add ideas, then move on to role plays about bystander action (Figure 6.2).

Maya's dilemma

Maya's "best friends" had ignored her all year. One September day, they came running over, out of the blue, and were the friendliest they had been since year 4. They started chatting to her, and she was excited. Could all the troubles be over? They told her they were going to the pool on the weekend, and she could join them. Maya felt a huge wave of happiness and relief wash over her. All the drama was over. But was it? After some chit-chat, they asked her what she thought of the boy standing alone next to the school canteen wall. She shrugged her shoulders, and a sick feeling came into her tummy. They asked, "Don't you think he's weird?" She froze. What was happening? Everything went from friendly to mean and fast. She knew they wanted her to join in, as they said a bucket load of mean things about this poor boy who'd never done anything to hurt anyone. Maya's parents had always taught her to be kind, no matter what. "Let's ask him why he's always alone!" perked up the "boss lady" of the group. Everyone happily chimed in, "Yes!" Maya froze again, and before she knew it, they grabbed her hand and pulled her along. She watched and said nothing as they taunted this poor boy, his eyes welling up with tears, his hands sweating, his skin red hot with fear. She didn't join in with words, but let them keep being mean…She didn't ask them to stop…She didn't walk away…She cared more about fitting in with them than doing what was right…

After school, Maya apologised to him, explaining that he didn't deserve what happened. He was silent, and she understood.

Ask your students: What might have been going on under the surface here? Why would she allow that kind of cruelty to happen without saying something? Why do kind people sometimes act meanly?

Invite everyone to reflect on a time they wished they'd acted differently with a friend. Remind them that mistakes are human—learning and moving forward matter.

Share the dos and don'ts of being a bystander poster.

Creating an "it's never cool to be cruel" school culture

Schools must take a zero-tolerance stance on bullying, as young people thrive in cultures where kindness prevails (Jin & Phusee-orn, 2024). Bullying is learned, but can be unlearned with clear expectations (Bear, 2020).

Bullying destroys confidence and well-being. It only takes away—it never gives.

The way forward is to build school and family cultures of kindness with zero tolerance for bullying. The next challenge is changing culture, especially in schools with so many voices and values.

The Cambridge dictionary definition of culture

If we turn to the Cambridge dictionary definition of culture, we find that culture is 'the way of life, especially the general customs and beliefs, of a particular group of people at a particular time.

Research shows that inclusive, emotionally supportive classrooms boost social-emotional development, self-regulation, academic success, and mental health, while reducing anxiety and behavioural issues (Bear, 2020; Jin & Phusee-orn, 2024; White et al., 2023).

SEE SOMEONE BEING HURT?

BE A HELPER, NOT A BYSTANDER

IT'S **NEVER OKAY** TO BE MEAN ON PURPOSE.

Here's how you can help if you see someone being treated badly:

✓ Do	Tell a grown-up or teacher right away.
✓ Do	If you feel safe, stand with the person being hurt. More friends nearby means less power for the bully.
✓ Do	If you feel safe, say, "That's not okay." out loud.
✓ Do	Move away and tell a teacher.
✓ Do	Tell an adult quietly if you need to stay safe.
✓ Do	Check in with the person who was hurt. Say, "Are you okay? Want to join us?"
✗ Don't	Join in or help the bully.
✗ Don't	Stand close to the bully.
✗ Don't	Laugh, agree, or do anything that makes it worse for the person being hurt.
✗ Don't	Start a fight.
✗ Don't	Try to fix everything yourself. Adults can help.

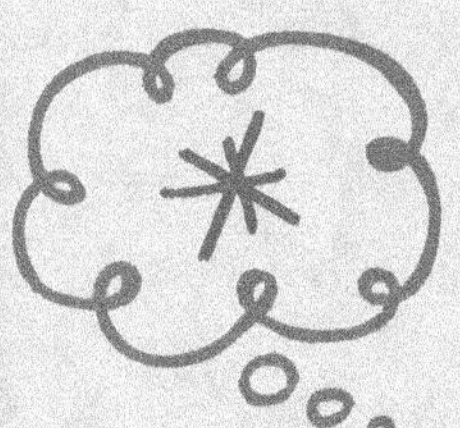

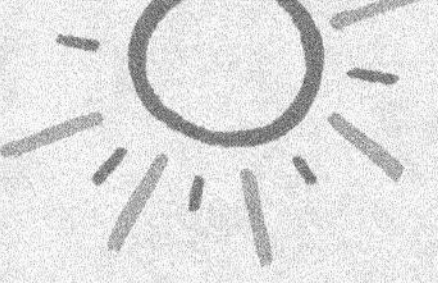

Jennings and Greenberg (2009) found that emotionally supportive classrooms foster students' social-emotional competence, which, in turn, enhances their engagement and learning. Zins et al. (2004) highlighted that social-emotional learning (SEL) programs, such as "The Friendship Blueprint," implemented in positive classroom settings, led to better mental health and academic outcomes. Hamre and Pianta (2001) found that students in classrooms with high levels of emotional support demonstrated stronger academic progress, particularly in early childhood education. Durlak et al. (2011) conducted a meta-analysis of SEL programs and found that students in positive classroom environments scored 11 percentile points higher in academic performance than those in less supportive settings.

A "way of life" blueprint for cultures of kindness, empathy, and connection (because it's never cool to be cruel).

Students now understand respectful relationships and can help shape your school's blueprint for safety and belonging.

Invite the group to complete a brief survey (I use SurveyMonkey) where they can be assured of their anonymity. Ideally, to change culture, every student in your school does this (and as mentioned in the introduction, every student is following "The Friendship Blueprint.")

Survey questions

Has anyone been mean to you on purpose at school? Yes/No

Do you want bullying (being mean on purpose) to stop at your school? Yes/No

If someone bullies you (is mean to you on purpose), do you want someone to come over and help you? Yes/No

Do you think parents and carers of bullies should be told about their child bullying (being mean on purpose)? Yes/No

Do you think there should be consequences for bullying (being mean on purpose) at your school? Yes/No

After collecting answers, share the results with your class. For younger students, adapt the survey for small-group discussion.

Share the results and have students create posters titled, "It's never cool to be cruel."

Include key statistics on the posters (e.g., most students want bullying to stop and support for those targeted).

Display the posters to show that bullying isn't tolerated and kindness is valued school-wide.

Kindness is never wasted; cruelty is never acceptable

Being kind isn't always easy, especially when you're frustrated or think you're right.

Random acts of kindness increase well-being for both giver and receiver (Layous et al., 2012).

Teaching kindness starts with adults modelling it. When we show empathy and kindness, children learn by watching.

Giving children opportunities to help and speak kindly fosters compassion. When they see us treat others gently, they internalise these skills. Kindness is uplifting and contagious—it ripples outward. Happier people spread positivity in their communities.

The heart collector game. (Empathy and Perspective Taking, Self-Awareness, Communication Skills)

Every kind or cruel action changes the strength of our hearts, and the hearts around us.

Show students how kindness builds connection and happiness, while cruelty damages both.

Give each student five paper hearts (or heart tokens, sticky notes, or hand-drawn hearts) to use during the activity.

Each heart represents emotional energy and a sense of belonging.

Designate one area temporarily as **Kindland** (a safe, kind zone) and another temporarily as **Meanland** (a space for unkind actions).

Explain that everyone starts with full hearts (five each), and their goal is to finish the game with as many hearts as possible, but *not by stealing*. They must *earn* hearts through kind acts.

Round 1. A kindness storm

Players move around the room and perform acts of kindness (real or symbolic), such as giving a compliment, helping someone up, or saying, "You can join us!"

Each time someone experiences or witnesses kindness, they *give their heart* to the person who was kind. After 3 minutes, pause and count the number of hearts.

Ask: "How do you feel right now?"

Round 2. A meanness test

Tell them that, just for one minute, you'll play a pretend version of what happens when people are *unkind on purpose*. Choose a few volunteers (or yourself) to act out mean or exclusionary behaviour (e.g., ignoring someone, whispering, saying "you can't play").

Anyone who witnesses unkindness *loses heart* because unkindness drains *everyone's* energy.

After one minute, stop immediately and collect the group.

Ask: "How did your body feel in that round?"
"What happened to your hearts?"
"Would you want to live in Meanland or Kindland?"

Round 3. A healing round

Kindness can repair hurt hearts. Players go around finding people who lost hearts and do something kind to help them earn one back. The goal is to ensure that *no one ends the game with fewer hearts than they started with*.

Debrief and reflection

Bring the group together for discussion or journalling:

"What did it feel like to lose a heart?"
"What did it feel like to get one back?"
"What can we learn about how kindness and cruelty affect people in real life?"

End the session with a simple statement like, "Kindness gives energy. Meanness drains it. Every choice you make changes the world around you."

A kindness quest. (Empathy and Perspective Taking, Self-Awareness, Communication Skills)

Perform intentional acts of kindness around the school, track them as a class, and reflect on the impact to build connection, empathy, and a sense of belonging. Create a large "Kindness Map" poster (or digital board) of the school with spaces for each classroom, common area, or student group. Provide plenty of stickers, stamps, or small tokens to mark completed acts.

Share the kindness quest ideas on your screen or point them out to the poster.

Introduce the "Kindness Map" in the classroom. Each time the class completes an act, they mark it on the map, showing how kindness spreads throughout the school.

Launch the quest across your school: Explain to students that the class is going on a "Kindness Quest," where every act of kindness adds power to the class's "Kindness Energy" (represented by filling in the map).

Collaborate and reflect: After completing the acts, ask your students the following questions:

Who did the act impact?

How did it make the class feel?

How did it make the person performing it feel?

Celebrate when the Kindness Map fills up with acts—reward the class with a small celebration.

Secret Kindness Week: Students perform acts of kindness anonymously, and the class guesses who is responsible for each act.

Expand school-wide by linking classrooms in a "Kindness Chain" poster or display.

Kindness quest ideas

Compliment a classmate on something they did well today.

Invite someone who usually plays alone to play with you at recess.

Write a positive note for a friend and leave it on their desk.

Ask a classmate how they are feeling and really listen.

Help a classmate with a task without being asked.

Share a snack or treat with a friend.

Say "thank you" to someone who helps you in class.
Give someone a high five or a fist bump for encouragement.
Share something you appreciate about a friend.
Sit with someone new at lunch.
Draw a picture for a friend to make them smile.
Share a classroom supply with someone who needs it.
Ask someone who hasn't been included to join your group project.
Share a joke with a friend to make them laugh.
Offer to carry something for a classmate.
Compliment someone on their handwriting, art, or work.
Include someone in a game you are playing.
Give someone a thumbs-up for trying their best.
Help a classmate clean up after an activity.
Write a short "You are awesome" note for someone and hand it to them secretly.
Say "thank you" to a teacher or staff member for something they do.
Leave a positive note for the principal, librarian, or office staff.
Compliment a teacher on their lesson today.
Smile and greet a staff member in the hallway.
Pick up something someone dropped and give it back politely.
Hold the door open for a teacher or staff member.
Give a staff member a thank-you card for helping the class.
Draw a "thank you" picture for the cleaner.
Offer to help set up or tidy a shared space in school.
Pick up litter in your classroom or school yard.
Organise a shared classroom space.
Water a classroom plant or help care for school greenery.
Write a kind message on the school whiteboard.
Help clean up the playground equipment after recess.
Draw a colourful sidewalk chalk message for others to see.
Put stray books back in the library or classroom shelves.
Help a younger student find their place in school.

Kindness rocks. (Self-Awareness, Communication Skills)

Creative expression improves well-being and community (Cohen, 2001). Have students paint rocks with positive messages and place them around the school.

Inclusion. (Empathy and Perspective Taking, Communication Skills, Self-Awareness)

Microaggressions among peers are common and hurtful. All children need belonging. Sometimes struggles at home or school lead to unkindness and exclusion, especially towards those seen as different. When microaggressions go unaddressed, their effects build up. Schools that value diversity and inclusion can reduce these issues (White et al., 2023).

Educators can create environments that highlight the benefits of diverse thinking, rather than expecting neurodivergent people to fit a neurotypical mould (White et al., 2023).

When families and schools don't teach genuine inclusion and appreciation for all kinds of minds, cruelty and exclusion can slip through. Children aren't born cruel; they can learn from the start to treat everyone with respect and openness, regardless of background or thinking style. That's the path to thriving communities.

Intentional cruelty damages children's well-being, self-esteem, and school engagement (Binfet & Passmore, 2017).

Belonging is crucial to well-being, and empathy encourages prosocial behaviour, such as inclusion (Zahn-Waxler et al., 1992).

Group discussion, microaggressions. (Empathy and Perspective Taking, Self-Awareness, Communication Skills)

Explain microaggressions simply using previous examples.

Refer to the following examples of microaggressions to increase awareness and understanding.

Ignoring someone's name or giving them a nickname because their real name is "too hard to say."

Assuming someone doesn't celebrate a holiday or know a song because of their culture or religion.

Speaking loudly or slowly to a child with an accent or speech difference.

Choosing only friends who "look like me" or leaving someone out of a game because "they're not in our group."

Laughing when a child brings a lunch that smells or looks different.

Interrupting or talking over someone who communicates differently or takes longer to respond.

Making comments about someone's hair, skin colour, or clothing in a way that sounds like a joke.

Not sitting next to a child who uses a wheelchair or sensory tools.

Assuming a child with autism, ADHD, or anxiety can't join in or won't understand.

Failing to include someone in play or conversation and saying, "I didn't mean to do that, it just happened."

Deeply understanding microaggression and exclusion to increase perspective and empathy

Start by summarising what microaggression and inclusion mean at your school. You might say something like:

> Sometimes people forget to notice people who are different from them, their names, foods, or how they play. That can make them feel invisible, like they don't belong or matter at our school. We're going to learn how to notice and include everyone. It's all our jobs to do our part in making the world a kinder and happier place for all.

Offer the following examples (or previous ones) of microaggressions and allow time for discussion after each one.

Ask, "How might that person feel?" and "What kind of action could happen instead?" to build empathy and understanding.

Examples of microaggressions

Ignoring someone because they don't look or sound like your friends.

Laughing when someone's lunch looks or smells different.

Saying, "Your name is too hard, so I'll call you something else."

Leaving someone out of a game because they play differently.

Pretending not to hear someone who speaks softly or takes time to find words.

Good reasons to delete microaggressions and make our school a kind and inclusive place

Kindness makes everyone feel safe and ready to learn

Kindness and inclusion foster psychological safety, enabling everyone to feel secure and learn better (Bear, 2020).

Inclusion builds stronger friendships

Including everyone, regardless of background, brings diverse perspectives and helps groups solve problems (White et al., 2023).

Being kind helps your body feel good

Acts of kindness release oxytocin and serotonin, boosting happiness and calm—a phenomenon known as the "helper's high" (Layous et al., 2012).

Inclusion helps us see the world more clearly

Listening to and including diverse peers strengthens empathy and perspective-taking (Zins et al., 2004).

Kind and inclusive schools change the world

Kindness and inclusion create a ripple effect, inspiring others and spreading positive culture school-wide (Layous et al., 2012).

Role-play rewind. (Empathy and Perspective Taking, Communication Skills)

Act out one microaggression scenario twice, the *Unkind* way and the *Kind* rewind way. Then ask your students, "Which ones help everyone feel like they belong?"

Kindness Promise. (Self-Awareness, Empathy and Perspective Taking)

Hand out journals or paper to allow some time for students to write or draw, reflecting on what they've learnt about microaggressions and the necessity for kindness. Ask them to take a moment to look inside their hearts and think about how being mean on purpose can spread quickly in a school, and how kindness can, too. Choosing kindness makes us all happier.

Invite students to make a self-leadership agreement with themselves to choose using their strengths, character, and values to show kindness each day.

Neurodivergence and inclusion

The world has improved. Diverse, inclusive schools and workplaces are no longer just a "nice idea"; including the strengths, voices, and experiences of neurodivergent people is a recognised necessity that enables the creation of deep, interesting, intelligent, and thriving societies. There is still a long way to go, but it is better than it was.

When I began my work in the 1990s with neurodivergent people, awareness, let alone understanding, was minimal. I remember the excitement when I started my dream job, teaching educators and students to notice, appreciate, and utilise the strengths of neurodivergent people.

I thought teaching friendship and compassion skills, along with showcasing the strengths and advantages of neurodivergent minds in schools, would naturally lead to inclusive, happy, and thriving school communities. What I didn't realise in my youth and inexperience is how crucial every person in a school community is to impact a culture. Every student, parent, and educator needs to hear and understand the same message and be willing to try something new.

If inclusion isn't meaningful to everyone, especially adults who lead young people in families and schools, then there's no guarantee it will matter to children. Families, schools, and workplaces need to collaborate to establish clear expectations about what will and won't be tolerated in their respective cultures. The goal of creating psychologically safe communities is entirely fair, and you'd be hard-pressed to find anyone who doesn't seek it and feels safe and comfortable in it.

If the consequences for intentional cruelty towards diverse groups are not clear, then those who struggle to treat people respectfully won't learn the power of genuine, safe relationships, nor will they experience the joy and benefits of getting to know a broad range of personalities, cultures, thinking styles, and personal strengths. Social skills like inclusion, warmth, empathy, and supportive communication not only improve who we are but also help advance others. In the end, those who fail to develop the skills that foster psychological safety will be at a social disadvantage and may experience ongoing challenges in finding depth and meaning in their social relationships. Not being open-hearted and minded limits who you will get to know in your lifetime and how much you will learn and grow as a person. Maintaining high expectations for kindness and inclusion is a vital ingredient for a happy and peaceful community.

When neurodivergent people are appreciated for the unique strengths they bring into communities, they experience the psychological safety to be themselves, and they can utilise these strengths instead of putting so much of their energy into coping with the isolation and lack of respect, and instead put it towards being authentic and bringing their much-needed contributions to the school community and beyond.

Diverse thinking and communication styles strengthen the world in ways it could not grow if only neurotypical thinking and communication styles were brought to the table. Limiting ourselves to the voices and perspectives of people like us weakens us and puts a full stop where a comma belongs in our understanding of the world.

The great inclusion challenge. (Empathy and Perspective Taking, Communication Skills, Self-Awareness)

Let's make our school a place where everyone feels safe and knows they belong.

How to Play: Try to complete as many of these 10 challenges as you can this week. Notice how each act helps others feel seen, valued, and included.

Buddy up challenge

Invite a student who's often alone to join your game, group, or table. Everyone deserves a seat and a smile.

Listen and learn challenge

Ask someone about their culture, language, or family tradition, and really listen. You might learn something amazing.

Patience power challenge

Show extra patience and kindness when someone learns, moves, or communicates in a different way. Celebrate their effort, not just speed or style.

Celebrate differences challenge

Create a class display, poster, or presentation that highlights the diverse abilities, cultures, and strengths in your classroom.

Fair share challenge

Ensure that everyone gets a chance to speak, play, or lead, even if they're quiet, shy, or think differently.

Kind words challenge

Stand up gently but bravely if you hear unkind, biased, or teasing words. Say something like, "Hey, we include everyone here."

Support squad challenge

Offer help to someone who might need it, such as carrying a bag, explaining a task, or showing them where to go. Small actions = big impact.

Respect every family challenge

Remember that families come in all shapes and sizes. Include everyone when you talk about "parents," "homes," or "celebrations."

Neurodivergence appreciation challenge

Notice the strengths of classmates who think or learn differently. Maybe they're creative, focused, funny, or detail-oriented. Compliment that.

Reflection

At the end of the week, reflect or journal: How did being inclusive make me feel? How did it make others feel? What are some of your favourite ways to make sure everyone feels noticed, supported, and respected every day at school?"

The buddy bench. (Empathy and Perspective Taking, Communication Skills)

Set up a Buddy Bench in the school yard where students can go if they are feeling lonely or need a friend. Encourage other students to approach those sitting on the bench to offer kindness, friendship or include them in activities.

Key takeaways from Chapter 6

- Kindness is your superpower! Every small act can turn an ordinary day into something magical for you and your friends.
- Compassion is catching—when you show you care, others feel braver to do the same.
- Inclusion is like building a big, colourful team where everyone gets to play and shine.
- Notice and challenge unfair ideas (bias)—don't let them block new friendships or fun.
- Your words and actions are like seeds: plant kindness and watch a whole garden of happiness grow in your school!
- When you make a mistake or see someone left out, you always get another turn to be kind and help them feel they belong.
- The more you include others, the more awesome stories and ideas you'll discover together.
- Kindness, compassion, and inclusion are essential for fostering a sense of belonging and emotional safety in schools, benefiting both individuals and the broader community.
- Challenging personal bias and practising empathy help students broaden their friendships, appreciate diversity, and build stronger, fairer communities.
- Self-awareness and reflection enable students to understand their emotions, actions, and their impact on others, leading to more positive and respectful relationships.

Call to action

Let's make kindness and inclusion our school's superpower—every day, everywhere!

Celebrate differences by sharing stories and learning about each other's unique strengths.

Spot acts of kindness and give out "Kindness Hero" awards (stickers, certificates, high-fives).

Speak up when you see unfairness or someone left out—your voice matters!

Invite your family, teachers, and the whole school to join in kindness quests and challenges.

Decorate your classroom with a "Kindness Pledge"—everyone signs it and adds what kindness means to them.

References

Bear, G. G. (2020). *Improving school climate: Practical strategies to reduce behaviour problems and promote social and emotional learning*. Routledge. https://www.routledge.com/Improving-School-Climate-Practical-Strategies-to-Reduce-Behavior-Problems-and-Promote-Social-and-Emotional-Learning/Bear/p/book/9780815346401

Binfet, J.-T., & Passmore, H.-A. (2017). Teachers' perceptions of kindness at school. *The International Journal of Emotional Education*, 9(1), 37–53. https://files.eric.ed.gov/fulltext/EJ1137976.pdf

Cohen, G. D. (2001). *The Creative Age*. William Morrow paperbacks. https://www.amazon.com.au/Creative-Age-Awakening-Potential-Second/dp/0380976846

Durlak, J. A., Weissberg, R. P., Dymnicki, A. B., Taylor, R. D., & Schellinger, K. B. (2011). The impact of enhancing students' social and emotional learning: A meta-analysis of school-based Universal Interventions. *Child Development*, 82(1), 405–432. https://doi.org/10.1111/j.1467-8624.2010.01564.x

Hamre, K. B., & Pianta, C. R. (2001). Early teacher-child relationships and the trajectory of children's school outcomes through eighth grade. *Child Development*, 72. https://www.sciepub.com/reference/67623

Hosoda, K. K., & Estrada, M. (2024). The influence of kindness on academics' identity, well-being and stress. *PLoS One*, 19(10), e0312269–e0312269. https://doi.org/10.1371/journal.pone.0312269

Jennings, P. A., & Greenberg, M. T. (2009). The Prosocial classroom: Teacher social and emotional competence in relation to student and classroom outcomes. *Review of Educational Research*, 79(1), 491–525. https://doi.org/10.3102/0034654308325693

Jin, S., & Phusee-orn, S. (2024). Exploring the influential factors on positive bystander behavior in school bullying among middle school students in Chongzuo, China. *Journal of Education and Learning*, 14(2), 239. https://doi.org/10.5539/jel.v14n2p239

Layous, K., Nelson, S. K., Oberle, E., Schonert-Reichl, K. A., & Lyubomirsky, S. (2012). Kindness counts: Prompting prosocial behavior in preadolescents boosts peer acceptance and well-being. *PLoS One*, 7(12), e51380. https://doi.org/10.1371/journal.pone.0051380

White, J., McGarry, S., Falkmer, M., Scott, M., Williams, P. J., & Black, M. H. (2023). Creating inclusive schools for autistic students: A scoping review on elements contributing to strengths-based approaches. *Education Sciences*, 13(7), 709. https://doi.org/10.3390/educsci13070709

Zahn-Waxler, C., Radke-Yarrow, M., Wagner, E., & Chapman, M. (1992). Development of concern for others. *Developmental Psychology*, 28(1), 126–136. https://doi.org/10.1037/0012-1649.28.1.126

Zins, E. J., Weissberg, P. R., Wang, C. M., & Walberg, J. H. (2004). *Building academic success on social and emotional learning: What does the research say?*. Corwin Press. https://us.corwin.com/en-us/nam/building-academic-success-on-social-and-emotional-learning/book227013

Making things better when friendships go wrong

> While friendship disagreements are inevitable, when young people know how to genuinely repair hurt, trust rebuilds, and friendships are given a precious second chance.

The adventure begins: Your friendship quest

Imagine you're a friendship explorer on a quest! Every adventure has tricky moments—misunderstandings, miscommunications, and even feeling left out. But guess what? These challenges are your chance to level up your skills—like empathy, kindness, and teamwork. In this chapter, you'll learn how to be a true friendship hero: taking responsibility, showing real empathy, apologising with courage, and rebuilding trust. Get ready to discover how every conflict can become an opportunity for growth, helping you and your friends become closer and stronger than ever.

Misunderstandings and conflict are a normal part of friendship (Hymel et al., 2018). When handled with self-awareness, compassion, and respect, these moments help build communication, empathy, compromise, and trust (Durlak et al., 2011). This chapter teaches students to take responsibility, show real empathy, apologise sincerely, and rebuild trust. By exploring common causes, misunderstandings, miscommunications, and exclusion, children learn how empathy and kindness resolve issues.

DOI: 10.4324/9781003617570-7

The goal: help young people see conflict as a natural, constructive part of relationships.

Setting the scene

Different opinions and communication styles often lead to conflict, especially as children develop emotional regulation and empathy (Collaborative for Academic, Social, and Emotional Learning [CASEL], 2020). With supportive adults, these moments foster self-awareness and growth. In cases of intentional cruelty or toxicity, ending the friendship—with guidance—may be best.

Children need chances to practice communication, emotional regulation, empathy, and respect to build social-emotional well-being (Durlak et al., 2011).

Distinguishing bullying (intentional, repeated cruelty) from typical friendship squabbles is essential (Primrose, 2025). Intervening too quickly can sometimes end relationships that could have grown stronger with respectful communication and problem-solving.

Self-awareness and a willingness to restore trust and acknowledge mistakes show maturity in friendships. Expressing genuine regret and empathy focuses on the impact, demonstrating honesty and accountability rather than defensiveness.

Active listening and asking how to make things right fosters respect, understanding, and a desire to repair and move forward.

Meaningful behavioural changes and allowing space for healing show commitment to the relationship.

This chapter supports educators in helping students reflect on and improve their relationships, empowering them to take responsibility and understand the reasons behind it.

Observing the skills in action

Get ready for a real-life friendship mystery! Read the following case study to your students, and imagine you're detectives trying to solve the puzzle together.

Case study: The scooter mix-up mystery

Ellie and Jamila loved racing scooters. One day, Jamila's scooter crashed, and she got hurt. Ellie called out, "Hurry up, slowpoke!" Jamila felt hurt and walked home alone (Goleman, 1995).

Ellie didn't mean to be unkind, but didn't realise her words hurt. That night, she felt uneasy, remembering her dad's advice: listen if your heart whispers something isn't right.

The next morning, Ellie saw Jamila alone at school, but was too nervous to apologise and ran away. Jamila felt even more hurt and alone (Durlak et al., 2011).

Recess and lunch passed in silence. Jamila was tempted to talk to others, but remembered that last time she did, it made things worse and led to a lost friendship.

Jamila took a deep breath and remembered her teacher's words:

"When we break something between friends, kindness, courage, and care help make it better."

Jamila wished Ellie would apologise first, but decided to be brave. She realised saying sorry is hard, and Ellie might be scared too.

Jamila took a deep breath, approached Ellie, and said, "I miss you." Ellie hugged her, apologised, and asked, "How can I make it better?" Jamila shared her feelings, and Ellie promised to do better.

Something inside Jamila shifted. Ellie wasn't just saying sorry to make the problem go away; she *meant it*. Jamila quietly said, "It really hurt my knee and my feelings." Ellie nodded. "I want to make things better. Maybe we can walk our scooters together today?" Jamila thought about it, and then she smiled. A small smile at first, then a bigger one. "Okay", she said.

That afternoon, they met outside Ellie's house and walked their scooters side by side, laughing again, but this time they rode slower. The water from the lake along their street sparkled like a mirror, as if the lake itself was smiling. This was a big step for both. Talking about it wasn't as uncomfortable as they both thought it would be, and it solved everything out in the open, nice and quick. They were closer than ever before, and they had proof that silence can make everything worse, just as it had for Roxanne and Jamila the year before.

Educator reflection

Do your students manage conflict well?

What skills do they need to practise?

Are you aware when students are having conflicts?

Do children in your class tend to manage conflict well?

What skills seem to be missing in the children who struggle most with conflict and conflict resolution?

Do you tend to know when your students conflict with each other?

Student reflection

How did Jamila show courage?

What would you do in her place?

What lesson from the story can you use?

What do you think about Jamila's reaction to Ellie not waiting for her after the fall?

If you were Jamila, what would you have done to work through the problem?

What idea from the case study do you like best that you could find useful?

Making things better: When things go wrong, make it right

After hearing Jamila and Ellie's story, invite everyone to imagine themselves as friendship superheroes. Remind students that even superheroes have disagreements, and that's totally normal! (Hymel et al., 2018). It takes courage to see things from someone else's point of view (CASEL, 2020). Working through tricky times is what makes friendships super strong. Practise the following super skills to help fix problems together, and display the "When things go wrong, make it right" poster to keep these ideas in sight! (Figure 7.1).

FRIENDSHIP PROBLEMS?

HERE'S HOW TO BOUNCE BACK AND MAKE THINGS RIGHT.

1 **Calm down first, take deep breaths and wait until you feel calm.**

Take deep breaths, move your body if needed, and wait until you feel calm. Take slow, deep breaths and move your body if needed, calm minds make wise choices.

2 **Stick to the facts, ask yourself what really happened. Don't guess or exaggerate.**

Don't guess or exaggerate.
What really happened?
Don't guess or make it bigger than it is.

3 **Own your part, admit what you did. Don't blame or make excuses.**

Admit your part—don't blame or make excuses.

4 **Think about the impact, notice how your actions made your friend feel.**

Notice how your actions affected others. Show you care about their feelings. Notice how it affected you and your friend. Show you care about their feelings!

5 **Show you care, imagine being in their shoes and use kind words or actions.**

Imagine being in their shoes. Use kind words or actions that would help you if you were them. Imagine how your friend feels—what might help them?

6 **Say sorry and ask, "How can I make things better?" Listen and do what you promised.**

"How can I make things better?" Listen, and do what you promise. Use words or actions that would help you if you were in their place.

Ask: "How can I make things better?" Then listen and try your best! This shows you're taking responsibility and want to make things better.

7 **Give your friend time and space if they need it. Everyone heals at their own pace.**

Let your friend have time if they need it before talking more. Do what you promised—actions speak louder than words!

8 **Show with your actions that you mean it, keep your promises and do better next time.**

Words alone may not be enough. Show with your actions that you really mean it.

9 **Learn for next time, mistakes help you grow.**

Everyone makes mistakes—learn and grow so you don't repeat them!

Friendship fixers: Try-it-out role plays

Give students a chance to practise resolving friendship conflicts using these short scenarios.

Keep the poster visible to help students work through the following role plays.

Role-play each scenario in two ways: first, as the problem; then, as the solution. Practise both sides to see how resolution feels.

Conflict resolution

Roles: One student is a friend with a problem, the other tries to help resolve it.

Your friend borrowed your toy but forgot to return it. Now they are avoiding you.

The first student shares their feelings. The other listens, shows empathy, and suggests ways to make things better (e.g., "I feel upset because I wanted to play with it. Can we find a way to make it right?").

After each role play, discuss what worked and how everyone felt. Emphasise listening, empathy, and compromise.

Case study challenge: The forgotten invite!

Two friends are planning a game at recess and forget to invite their class-mate. The classmate overhears and feels hurt.

Roles: Friends planning, hurt classmate.

Resolution prompt: How could the friends include them now? What could the hurt classmate say to let them know how they feel?

Case study challenge: The soccer ball standoff!

Two children want to use the same soccer ball. Both grab it at once and argue.

Roles: Two children wanting the ball.

Resolution prompt: How could they share or take turns? What's a fair solution?

Case study challenge: The secret spill!

A child shares something private with their friend. Later, the friend tells others, and the first child feels betrayed.

Roles: Secret-sharer, friend who shared it, classmate who overheard.
Resolution prompt: How can the friend make it right? What could the child do to rebuild trust?

Case study challenge: The group project showdown!

In a small group, one child wants to do things one way, while another insists on their own idea.

Roles: Group members with different ideas.
Resolution prompt: How can they compromise or combine ideas so everyone feels included?

Case study challenge: The game rule rumble!

During a game, two children argue over which rule is correct.

Roles: Two players, optional referee.
Resolution prompt: How could they calmly discuss or vote on the rule? Could they agree on a new rule before continuing?

Questions to ask students that don't interfere with the natural process of conflict resolution

Support children as they learn independent problem-solving, but step in when emotional regulation or skills are lacking. Avoid group discussions if there's a power imbalance—sometimes, it's better to speak with each child separately to prevent further problems.

Let students know disagreements are normal everywhere. Understanding others' feelings and opinions is essential. If emotions are too big or problems too hard, encourage asking for help.

Share the following reflection framework and invite students to comment on and tweak it to suit your school culture.

Speak with each child privately and let them know you're there to help, not to blame. Ask open-ended questions to guide reflection.

Questions

Tell me more about what happened.
How did you feel at the time?
How do you think your friend felt when that happened?
What do you think could have been different if you had done it another way?
If you were your friend, how would you feel about yourself?
What can you do next time to stop feelings from being hurt?

These questions encourage empathy and self-awareness. Adjust them as needed. Give time for reflection and support reconnection in a caring way.

Knowing when to stop

Emotional dysregulation and impulsivity can cause children to go too far with a joke or disruptive behaviour, even after others ask them to stop. Knowing when to stop is hard for those who struggle with impulse control and social awareness, but it's an essential skill for confidence and healthy friendships.

Teaching this skill with a playful quiz helps make a tricky topic less embarrassing.

Quiz: Time to stop or not? (Self-Awareness, Communication Skills)

Have students listen to each scenario and use thumbs up for a clear signal to stop, thumbs to the side for a mixed signal, and thumbs down if everything is fine. Discuss each scenario together.

You're copying your friend as they groom their hair. They tell you to "quit it."
You're laughing loudly at your friend's joke. It's so loud that people at another table are looking. Someone at that table looks at you and starts laughing loudly, staring right at you and sounding like you.
You're asking a friend for a bite of their hot dog. They've promised to leave you some at the end. You keep sniffing the hot dog and saying how yummy it looks as they eat. They turn their body away and sigh.

You and your best friend are in the middle of a laughing fit. They are laughing so hard, and say, "stop, stop being so funny," and keep laughing with you.

You're commenting honestly about our friend's project that they asked for your opinion on. You think it's bad. You give honest, straight-up feedback, and your friend says, "Wow, thanks, that's made me feel great about myself. Do you have anything else you'd like to add? This is super helpful."

Knowing when to stop: Role plays (Communication Skills, Empathy, Perspective Taking)

Divide students into pairs for each role play. Encourage them to use the sample responses or create their own, using these prompts:

"How does it feel when someone keeps doing something when you've asked them to stop?"

"What's the easiest, kindest way to ask someone to stop?"

"If someone asks you to stop, what's the best way to respond?"

The tapping pencil

The pencil tapper: Child taps pencil continually.

Peer response: "Hey, that tapping is making it hard for me to concentrate. Can you stop, please?"

Tapper: "Oh, sorry. I didn't realise. I'll stop." The

Learning focus: Noticing the request and stopping without arguing.

The copycat

Silly talker: Repeats every word in a silly voice.

Peer response: "I don't like it when you copy me. Please stop."

Silly talker: "Okay, I'll stop. I thought it was funny, but I don't want to annoy you."

Learning focus: Recognising that jokes are only enjoyable if both people are laughing.

The ball hog

Ball hog: Keeps dribbling and won't pass.

Peer response: "We all want a turn. Can you share the ball, or we'll go play something else."

Ball hog: "You're right. I'll pass it now; your turn."
Learning focus: Recognising that not sharing can cause others to lose interest.

The too-close shadow

Follower: Follows closely, mimicking every move.
Peer response: "I need some space right now. Please stop following me."
Learning focus: Respecting personal boundaries and adjusting behaviour.
Follower: "Got it. I'll give you space."

The joke that never ends

Joker: Tells the same joke over and over.
Peer response: "That was funny the first time, but can we talk about something else now?"
Joker: "Okay, I'll stop. Thanks for telling me."
Learning focus: Picking up when laughter has stopped and moving on.

The singing voice

Singer: Sings loudly while the group is trying to work.
Peer response: "We can't focus with you singing. Can you save that for later?"
Singer: "Sure, I'll stop singing so we can get the work done."
Learning focus: Choosing the right time and place for silliness.

The shoulder poke

Poker: Keeps poking their friend's shoulder.
Peer response: "Please don't poke me. If you want my attention, just say my name."
Learning focus: Using words instead of repeated actions.
Poker: "Oh, okay. Next time I'll just call your name."

Knowing when to stop: Student reflection

Together as a class or in small groups, extend knowledge through the following questions:

"Why might something feel funny at first but not later?"
"How would it feel to be copied? How would it feel to stop?"

"How can you notice when people are getting frustrated with your behaviour?"
"Why is personal space important?"
"How do you know when you're too close to someone?"
"What are some signs that people have had enough of a joke?"
"What's a better way to keep the fun going without repeating?"
"Why might singing be okay sometimes but not other times?"
"How can you tell when it's the right time to be silly?"
"Why might poking be annoying even if it's not meant to hurt?"
"What are better ways to get someone's attention?"

Tuning in with others and knowing when to stop through self-awareness and self-regulation

Helping children develop self- and social-awareness lets them self-regulate without constant feedback. Over-excitement or not knowing when to stop can disrupt others' enjoyment and sense of safety. Compassion is important for those who find this hard, but not teaching these skills can lead to isolation.

Game: The fun-o-meter

Creating cultures of WE instead of ME for a RIPPLE effect of self-awareness, empathy, and perspective-taking.

This game provides opportunities to practice self-regulation, empathy, and flexible thinking. Recognising when you've gone too far and aren't being considerate of others, and registering other people's signals that it's time to slow down, stop, or change, is an essential social skill that benefits everyone involved.

Tell students that the fun-o-meter game is about balancing fun with respect for others' comfort. What's funny to one person can be too much for someone else. Paying attention to everyone's comfort is part of a kind school culture.

Create clear visual zones, sensory cues, and scripts for self-regulation and repair. Read and display the following poster to guide students through before you start the game (Figure 7.2).

WE NOT JUST ME COMMUNITY IS POWERFUL

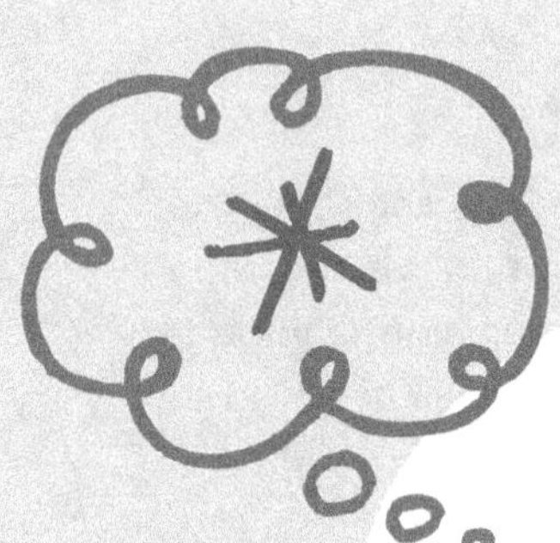

GREEN ZONE

Fun for everyone. Keep playing, everyone's happy.

AMBER ZONE

Fun for some, not all. Change things to make it better for everyone.

RED ZONE: STOP

If most aren't having fun, help fix it together.

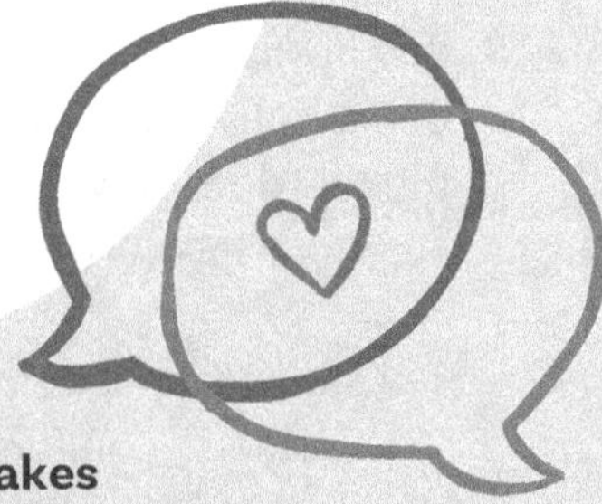

No matter the zone, everyone makes mistakes, let's always try again and be kind. In a WE school, everyone grows in kindness, empathy, and forgiveness. Even one kind act can make a big change.

Let's begin.

(As this game can get loud, remember to offer noise-cancelling headphones, soft lighting, or calming music between rounds, and fidget tools for children who need to regulate themselves during discussions.)

Introduce the fun zones

"Sometimes what's fun for you might feel too much for someone else. This game helps us notice when our fun is in the green zone, and when we might need to stop or slow down."

Create a fun zone wheel: Have students cut out a circle, divide it into green, orange, and red, and attach a moving arrow. Each keeps their own as a reminder. Reinforce the idea of "WE, not ME" and the ripple effect of kindness.

Part one of the Fun-O-Meter game: Fun detectives role play

How to play: Invite a child or a pair to stand in front of the group and do something fun for 30 seconds (make a silly sound, do a funny dance, or leap into a funny movement).

Quietly, students hold up their Fun-O-Meter rating it: Green, Orange, or Red, which may change during the 30-second role play.

Ask the student at the front to notice the colour zones their peers display. If most show red or orange, they should reset or stop. Remind them to respond kindly to feedback and practise phrases like, "Thanks for letting me know, I'll stop now," or "Sorry, how can I make it better?"

After each turn, ask: "What clues did you notice that told you it was still fun, or not fun anymore?"

Support students who receive orange or red feedback by helping them avoid feeling defensive and reminding them it's a role play for learning together. Support peers to respect individual differences and developmental stages, pointing out the **WE** of change where everyone works together, supporting personal bests by showing kindness, empathy, and compassion for those who struggle, not criticism or judgment.

Reiterate the challenge of self-awareness when you're in the thick of fun. Compassionately help students understand self-check-ins on how their bodies feel when they're excited, and how to notice other people's responses and comfort, pointing out that everyone has a right to feel safe at school.

Part two of the "Fun-O-Meter," game: A tune-in challenge

In small teams, students create a 30-second fun routine, such as a rhythm, a movement, or a short scene. For the entire thirty seconds, their goal is to keep their routine in the **Green Zone for everyone**. Peers hold up their Fun-O-Meters to help the performers know when to adjust by slowing down, resetting, or quieting down where needed.

After each performance or turn, run a gentle reflection circle asking the performers:

"When did you feel most excited?"
"When did you notice someone might not be having fun anymore?"
"What did you do to make it better?"

Moving forward, include the Fun-O-Meter as a daily classroom tool that serves as a visual reminder to strike a balance between personal excitement and mutual respect, and to remember the power of WE. You might also like to create personal "Regulation Kits" (small boxes with fidgets, pictures, breathing tools).

Emotional regulation and the power of a big, deep, and calming breath before you speak. (Self-Awareness, Conflict Resolution, and Problem Solving)

Big feelings can make our thoughts race and lead to regretful reactions. When friendships go wrong, the pain can be intense, so it's easy to react without thinking.

Slow, deep breathing oxygenates the brain, triggering calm, and releasing rational thinking. Often, in the heat of the moment, when emotions run high, there is little or no space between an action and a reaction. Children need to know how receptive the mind is to the power of a long, deep breath, placed in that small but mighty space between an event and our response, to trigger emotional regulation and rational perspective.

Regulated breathing reduces emotional flare-ups and helps children solve problems respectfully without adult intervention. Breathing deeply after an upset moves us from defensiveness to calm problem-solving.

Invite students to share helpful breathing techniques, then practise the ideas from the "Breathe big, think bigger" poster together (Figure 7.3).

BREATHE BIG
THINK BIGGER

CALM DOWN AND YOUR BEST IDEAS WILL SHINE.

Take a few big, deep breaths before you respond to a problem. When you are calm, it's easier to solve problems.

HOW TO BREATHE:

Breathe in for 5 seconds through your nose, hold for 5, then breathe out slowly for 5–10 seconds.

Breathe in through your nose and out through pursed lips slowly, as many times as you need.

Try 4-7-8 breathing
Breathe in for 4, hold for 7, breathe out for 8.

Breathe in slowly
When your lungs are full, sip in a little more air, then hold and release after 5–10 seconds.

Finger breathing
Trace your fingers as you slowly breathe in and out. Imagine your breath is a gentle wave.

That tiny space between an event and your response is best filled with a slow, deep breath. Remind students that friendship problems can trigger big emotions, and belonging helps us feel safe. Encourage them to breathe before reacting (Figure 7.4).

Be realistic and fair when teaching this skill to young people. Self-regulation and mindfulness are not easy when you're in social pain. Just think of how many adults are unable to do this (even with fully developed brains).

While it's up to us to model and teach the skill, as well as support them in remembering and practising it, we need to consider their age and developmental capabilities and not be too hard on them for forgetting. Childhood is the time to practice these skills, ready for the big, wide world of adult relationships.

Role plays that start with a breath, then thinking, and finally, a solution. (Self-Awareness, Conflict Resolution and Problem Solving, Empathy and Perspective Taking)

Divide the group into three for the following role plays. Their goal is for two people to engage with the problems below, practice breathing before speaking or acting, and then think out loud to demonstrate that they are switching on empathy and perspective before attempting to solve the issue.

Allow students to have one narrator who comments on what is happening. For example,

Narrator: "Sima starts with a slow breath…oh, she's going to need a few of those. In and out she goes. Now that she can think straight, she asks herself, "Is winning this argument more important than our friendship?" and then she tells her friend, and the problem is solved. Let's give a cheer for Sima!

Role plays

Changing the rules in the middle of a game

Two friends are playing a board game. One child suddenly changes the rules to win.

The other child feels cheated and frustrated. Show how the "rule-changer" reacts when challenged and how the other child could respond (after taking

FRIENDSHIP PROBLEMS?

HERE'S HOW TO FEEL BETTER AND FIX IT.

Pause and take big, deep breaths before you respond. When you are calm, it's easier to solve problems.

Use your breath to calm down, then find a kind way to fix things.

1 **Breathe deeply: slow in, slow out.**

Kindness returns after a few deep breaths. Breathe until you feel calm and ready to talk.

2 **Check in with yourself, are you ready to talk kindly?**

Still mad? Keep breathing or move your body to let the feelings out.

3 **Think, what's your friend's side of the story?**

How will your friend feel if you yell, push, or say something mean?

Is there a kinder way to tell your friend how you feel?

Would you like it if they did the same to you?

4 **Take action, work it out with your friend.**

Ask your friend, "How can I make things better?" or "Can we work this out?"

Show your friend you're sorry—write a note, make a card, or say it out loud. Notice what helps them feel better.

5 **Move forward, everyone makes mistakes and can try again.**

Everyone messes up sometimes, especially with big feelings. Learn, do better, and ask an adult for help if you need it.

The Friendship Blueprint™ by Madhavi Nawana Parker • www.madhavinawanaparker.com.au

a breath). They could walk away, negotiate, or calmly state something like, "That's not fair, let's stick to the rules."

The unfair team picker

During recess sports, one child chooses teams and consistently picks their best friends first, leaving others to last. Someone feels left out and angry at always being chosen last.

Act out both perspectives (how it feels to be left until last, and how the chooser could be fairer).

The credit stealer

A group project is finished, but one child claims they did most of the work even though it was shared equally. The others feel upset that their hard work is being ignored. Demonstrate how the group can speak up kindly, without escalating an argument, and how the teacher might intervene.

The seat saver

A child puts their bag on a seat at lunch, saying it's for their friend who isn't there yet, even though another child wants to sit down. The waiting child feels excluded and angry.

Show how the seat saver could rethink fairness, and how the other child might calmly express, "I need somewhere to sit too."

The toy grabber

Two children are building a Lego creation. One suddenly snatches all the best pieces and won't share. The other child feels furious about their selfishness. Act out what happens if the upset child yells versus calmly saying, "We need to share so both our builds work."

The story twister

A child tells the teacher a story that makes another student look bad, even though they've changed the truth, so they don't get into trouble themselves. The accused child feels wrongly blamed and helpless. Show how the accused might defend themselves, how the teacher could listen fairly, and how honesty matters.

The group excluder

A group is creating a play during recess. One child says, "You can't join because we don't need you," even though they could easily include them. The excluded person feels rejected and angry. Explore how it feels for both sides and how the group might shift to be more inclusive.

The bragging winner

After winning a running race, a child boasts loudly, "I'm the best, you're all too slow," and won't let others enjoy the game. Other children feel annoyed, angry, and belittled.

Demonstrate how bragging hurts others, and then illustrate how to celebrate without putting others down.

Social awareness through empathy and kindness. (Empathy and Perspective Taking, Self-Awareness)

Noticing how others think and feel is a social skill that takes practice. Everyone learns at their own pace, but giving all students opportunities to practise can strengthen relationships and reduce misunderstandings.

The schoolyard provides countless opportunities for children to develop social awareness by observing and interacting with other people's character, values, and capabilities. It provides an ideal backdrop for diversity, different perspectives, and adaptability. Without these opportunities, children often lack the necessary practice to manage the discomfort of differing opinions and values and to transition through that discomfort into confidence and adaptability. Social awareness develops as children learn to notice and respectfully communicate their differing opinions, compromise when fair, and reach mutually respectful solutions for friendship challenges by considering the other person's experience as well as their own. Most people view their experiences through their own perspectives, values, and character. This can be limiting and leaves plenty of room for misunderstandings and flare-ups. Understanding that friendship is two-sided and being aware of each other's feelings is not only helpful but also kind and considerate.

Gently explain this skill to your students, noting that some may find it harder than others. Be supportive, kind, and patient (CASEL, 2020).

Game: Friendship glue and friendship eraser. (Self-Awareness, Empathy, and Perspective Taking)

Children often find friends with shared values (Hymel et al., 2018), but sometimes choose playmates out of loneliness or imbalance. "Friendship glue" are traits that hold friendships together; "friendship erasers" are what weaken them.

Share the following poster and hand out paper and markers for students to create their own friendship glue and eraser posters (Figure 7.5).

After students finish their posters, discuss which character traits strengthen or weaken friendships.

Empathy to help when Friendships go wrong. (Empathy and Perspective Taking)

Empathy, like social awareness, comes more naturally to some than others (Durlak et al., 2011). People show empathy in different ways and at different times.

Empathy, like kindness, is never wasted (Goleman, 1995). It calms emotions by helping us feel seen and valued. Everyone shows empathy differently, so it's important to separate **intent** from **impact**.

Discuss the "Empathy why, and empathy how" framework. Invite students to share their understanding. Teaching empathy supports social-emotional learning (CASEL, 2020).

Empathy why? Empathy how?

Why does empathy matter?

Empathy helps us step out of what is true for ourselves and step into what is true for someone else. Empathy strengthens friendships by seeing situations from our friends' eyes, not just our own. When we give (and receive) empathy and kindness, our brains release neurotransmitters like serotonin and dopamine, motivating us to take positive action. Empathy and kindness are nature's way of spreading joy, uplifting each other, and strengthening our community.

FRIENDSHIP GLUE & ERASERS

STICK TOGETHER WITH KINDNESS.

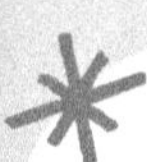

FRIENDSHIP GLUE

What Makes Friendships Stick

- Kindness
- Honesty
- Loyalty
- Empathy
- Fairness
- Friendliness
- Patience
- Sharing
- Listening
- Encouraging
- Smiling
- Compliments
- Warmth
- Respect
- Caring
- Forgiveness
- Gentleness
- Understanding
- Compassion
- Support
- Uplifting
- Giving

FRIENDSHIP ERASERS

What Breaks Friendships

- Meanness
- Lying
- Spreading rumours
- Laughing at others
- Setting someone up
- Talking behind backs
- Mean comments
- Discrimination
- Ignoring
- Hurting
- Not stopping when asked

GLUE STRENGTHENS, ERASERS WEAKEN. CHOOSE KINDNESS AND BE THE GLUE.

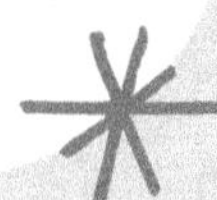

Empathy how

Empathy is feeling with someone, not just feeling for them.

Empathy is paying attention to what someone else feels and showing them kindness.

Empathy is trying to imagine what it's like to be another person and behaving towards them how you would like them to behave towards you.

Empathy is seeing the world through someone else's heart.

Empathy is listening with your heart as well as your ears.

Empathy is connecting your feelings to someone else's experience.

Game: Step into their shoes. (Empathy and Perspective Taking)

It's time to put their learning into action. Assign each child a character trait from the Friendship Glue poster to use during the Role-Play. Pair by pair, students role-play the problem using their assigned character trait to work through their problem. If you feel your students can handle it, allow one member of the pair to take on a character from the friendship eraser list, giving them an opportunity to be challenged by a difficult character trait.

Read out the following short social situations for your students to re-enact with the character trait they've been assigned.

A new student joins the class, looking nervous.

Your team loses a game on sports day.

Someone tells a joke that not everyone finds funny.

A friend forgets to invite you to their birthday.

Your friend freezes in fear just as they are called to collect an award during your school assembly.

Someone has just been bullied by some older students and can't stop crying.

A friend's pet rabbit has been lost for three days, and they are devastated.

One of your best friends is being intentionally mean to your new friend.

Your parents invited work friends over for dinner. Their children just came tearing through your personal things in your room and made a huge mess. You want them to stop.

You overheard your best friend talking about their birthday party this weekend. You ask them if they are doing anything for their birthday, thinking they will invite you. They tell you they aren't celebrating this year.

Act it out

Children role-play how their character trait would handle the situation. For example:

If they have *kindness*, they might offer comfort, say something kind, or do something thoughtful, without getting involved, being assertive, and so on. If they have a sense of *humour*, they might make a joke to break the ice or see the lighter side of things.
If they have *independence*, they might go off to do their own thing or express their thoughts, even if others disagree.

After the role-play, the rest of the group guesses which character trait each player was using.

> **Reflection circle. After the Role Plays, ask your students**
> How did different values lead to different choices?
> Was one way better than another? Or just different?
> How can understanding people's values and personalities help us get along better?

The same situation can be handled in many ways. Students learn that differences in values and personality enrich friendships and communities.

Intent and impact. (Self-Awareness, Empathy and Perspective Taking, Communication Skills)

Most children don't mean to upset others, but social mistakes happen as they learn. Emotions can make conflicts escalate quickly. It's important to show understanding, but also to be clear that even if the hurt wasn't intended, accountability and repair are needed. Learning to be accountable and make amends is vital for healthy relationships.

Understanding *intent* versus *impact* helps children take responsibility for their actions, even when they didn't mean harm. Gently show them that hurt has occurred and that making repairs matters. Every action creates a ripple effect.

Using empathy as a GPS, we can help guide students to notice and value each other's thoughts and feelings, so we can live our lives not only for ourselves but through the gift of friendships. The more we understand each other, the less likely we are to unintentionally hurt others.

The ripple game: Intention vs. impact

Materials: Paper "ripples" (large circles cut from paper), markers, and a ball (a soft foam ball works best).

Step 1: What's the difference?

Ask: "Have you ever said or done something that you didn't mean to be mean, but it still hurt someone's feelings?" Give a simple example, like: "If I say, 'Move over!' because I want to sit down, I might not mean to be rude, but the other person might feel like I don't care about them."

Intention = what you meant to do. **Impact** = how it made the other person feel.

Step 2: The ripple story

Place the paper ripples on the floor like a pond.

Stand in a circle and roll the ball into the "pond." Explain: "When we do something, even if we don't mean to hurt anyone, it can ripple out and affect others."

Encourage students to give examples, and prompt them with the ideas that follow if needed: I was trying to be funny (intention), but someone felt embarrassed (impact).

I wanted to win the game (intention), but I left someone out (impact).

I wanted to surprise my sister by redecorating her room while she was away (intention), but she was upset because I didn't ask and changed the way she liked it (impact).

I wanted to impress my teacher and show them I'd been listening, so I raised my hand for every question and answered it (intention). However, after a while, my classmates got frustrated with me for not giving anyone else a chance to answer (impact).

I wanted to help my friend improve their literacy skills (intention), but they were upset that I kept correcting them and pointing out their mistakes (impact).

I wanted the class to follow the rules and be safe (intention), but everyone got upset with me for telling the teacher they were being silly (impact).

After giving each example of intention, the speaker gently bounces the ball and lets it roll across the ripples, sharing the impact as a reminder that good intentions don't guarantee good outcomes.

Step 3: Fixing the ripples

As children learn to navigate the complex social world, they will inevitably make social blunders. Knowing how to make things better and keep moving forward together is an essential part of school and keeps the bridges between friends strong.

Ask your students: "If a ripple has gone out and hurt someone, what can we do?"

Ideas: Own up without being defensive and say sorry in a kind way. Check in with the person's feelings. Offer to make it better (play again, give space, invite them in, etc.). Reflect later, using empathy and kindness to help solidify your new skill.

Allow time to brainstorm repair ideas. Then, play repair together using the ripple story from earlier or the scripts that follow the reflection.

Step 4: Reflection

"Sometimes our intentions are good, but the impact can still hurt. That doesn't make us bad people, it just means we need to notice the ripple and take care of it with kindness and respect."

Intention vs impact role plays. (Empathy and Perspective Taking, Communication Skills).

Divide your class into pairs to practice role-playing their new knowledge.

The joke that hurt

Child A (intention): "I was just trying to be funny when I called you a silly name."

Child B (impact): "It made me feel embarrassed. I didn't like being laughed at."

Repair (A): "I'm sorry, I meant it as a joke, but I can see it hurt. I won't do that again."

Repair (B): "Thanks for saying sorry. I feel better."

The rushed grab

Child A (intention): "I just wanted the red pencil quickly."

Child B (impact): "It felt like you didn't care about me when you grabbed it out of my hand."

Repair (A): "I didn't mean to upset you. Next time I'll ask first."

Repair (B): "That would be better, thanks."

The playtime whoops

Child A (intention): "I wanted to win the game, so I ran ahead without waiting."

Child B (impact): "I felt left out when you didn't wait for me."

Repair (A): "I'm sorry. Let's start again, and I'll make sure to include you."

Repair (B): "Okay, I'd like that."

The loud comment

Child A (intention): "I wanted everyone to know I won."

Child B (impact): "I felt like you were rubbing it in, and that hurt my feelings."

Repair (A): "I didn't mean to upset you. Next time I'll celebrate in a way that doesn't hurt."

Repair (B): "Thanks. That helps."

The sharing slipped up

Child A (intention): "I was excited to tell others your secret because I thought it was funny."
Child B (impact): "It hurt me because I trusted you, and now, I feel embarrassed."
Repair (A): "I'm sorry. I won't share things that aren't mine to tell. I'll tell the people I shared your secret with that I did the wrong thing and I shouldn't have told them."
Repair (B): "Thanks. I'd appreciate that.

After each role play, pause and ask the group:

What was the intention?
What was the impact?
What respectful repair was made?

This reinforces that even good intentions can cause hurt, and repairing is what matters most.

Empathy and compassion through the loving kindness practice. (Self-Awareness, Empathy, and Perspective Taking)

I grew up with parents who loved this practice. When Dad passed away suddenly at 45, I was 10, and somehow, Mum kept this practice alive for us. She continued starting her day, wishing others well, even during the intensity of her own grief and suffering. This was one of my favourite things about her: always generous, always willing to help, and always able to give love. Whenever I had an upset with a friend, she would remind me to take a moment and reset with loving kindness. I'll be honest, there were times when this was the last thing I wanted to do, but as the years have passed, this practice has helped me immensely to stay hopeful, optimistic, and connected to what truly matters through the many ups and downs of my life. I will be forever grateful for this generous gift, and it's a joy to include it here.

Loving kindness practice

To get the most out of this (and anything that requires your students to be still for a while), remember to let them expend some energy first. Just two minutes of fun physical activity can help release any energy that otherwise interrupts our ability to pause and bring our mind's work into action. I'm always encouraging short movement breaks at the start and middle of each lesson, not just in preparation for these moments, but that short moment away from learning gives back in abundance.

When students return from movement, invite them to sit or lie down comfortably, dim the lights, and play gentle background music if desired. When everyone is ready, you can begin.

Breathe in, breathe out

Take a big, slow breath in… and let it out slowly.
Again, a big breath in… and slowly out.

Think of you

Put your hand on your heart. Say quietly in your mind:

"I'm happy. I'm healthy. I'm safe."
Smile as you think it.

Think of someone you love

Now, think of someone you truly love from your family or friends. Say quietly in your mind:

"I hope you're happy. I hope you're healthy. I hope you feel safe."

Think of someone you don't know well or maybe someone you're having trouble with

Think of someone you see sometimes but don't know very well or someone you are having trouble with.
   Say quietly in your mind:

"I hope you are happy. I hope you are healthy. I hope you feel safe."

Think of everyone in the world

Think of all the people everywhere, even children and animals far away.
   Say quietly in your mind:

"I hope everyone is happy. I hope everyone is healthy. I hope everyone feels safe."

Take one more breath

Take one last deep breath in… and let it out slowly.
Wiggle your fingers and toes, open your eyes, smile, and remember, you can
   share love with yourself and everyone around you.

*Mutual respect and compassionate solutions: Role plays. (Conflict
Resolution and Problem Solving, Empathy and Perspective Taking)*

Encourage students to work in pairs and come up with common friendship
dilemmas like arguing over who got out in a game, or who came up with an
idea first. Students take turns playing each side of the conflict so both sides
of the story can be explored.

Debrief: Discuss how hearing both sides helped them understand the conflict better. Encourage the children to think about how they can apply this
   strategy in real-life situations.

On the news

It's time to have some fun broadcasting a mock news reading from your
classroom. Allow for costumes, rehearsals, creativity, and, if possible, record
it. Invite students to create a news story in which they are interviewed by a
host eager to learn what happened between two friends and how compassion built a bridge between them, resolving everything. The host brings in a
friendship expert to suggest solutions. Show the following poster to help and
remind students to include the following skills from this chapter:

Take a breath in the small and mighty space between social pain and your
   response.
Intent and impact.
Compassion and empathy.
Stay in the green zone and know when to stop (Figure 7.6).

Saying sorry and moving forward (repair and reconnect) when things go wrong with friends

Many children struggle to apologise and take ownership of their actions.
They tell me how embarrassing it is for them to admit when they have

FRIENDSHIP GLITCH?

FIX IT TOGETHER, TEAMWORK MAKES IT BETTER.

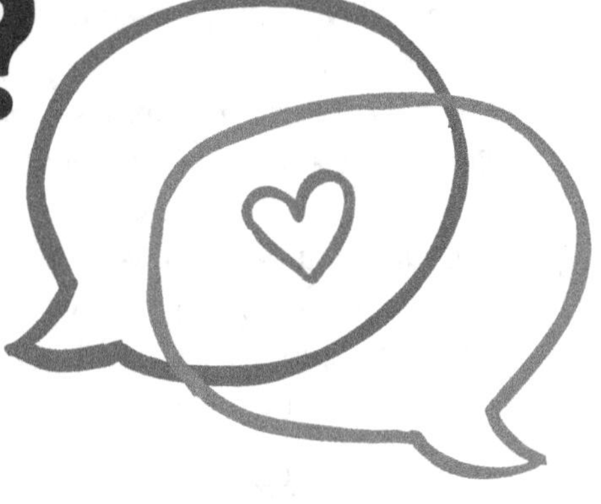

1 **Take a breath**, get ready to listen and speak kindly. Calm voices help.

2 **Ask questions and work together.** Ask, "How can we make this better or fair for both of us?"

3 **Listen and keep brainstorming.** Take turns, share ideas, or flip a coin if you can't agree.

4 **Pick a solution you both like.** If it doesn't work, try another idea together.

5 **Check in.** If it's not working, ask an adult for help. Being brave means asking for help.

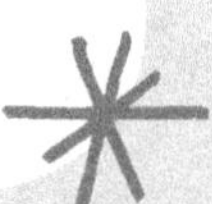
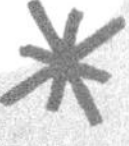

When you work together, everyone feels heard and respected, and your friendships get stronger.

The Friendship Blueprint™ by Madhavi Nawana Parker • www.madhavinawanaparker.com.au

done the wrong thing and how they worry it will make the person stop liking them. Normalising how we all make can help them see that everyone goes through these moments and feels uncomfortable about it. Remind your students that apologising is often difficult and challenging for most people. Avoiding an apology to avoid your own discomfort weakens your social-emotional intelligence and can make things worse.

For some children, apologising and taking responsibility can feel much harder than we expect. Rejection sensitivity is a well-established psychological trait, and there is growing empirical support that people (especially those with ADHD and neurodivergence) have heightened emotions when receiving feedback for doing the wrong thing and being asked to be accountable and take ownership (Ruwa, 2025). Emotions are disproportionately heightened whenever they make a mistake or are asked to take accountability, and they worry they have disappointed others or will be rejected by the people they love. For those who experience this sensitivity, apologising doesn't just mean "saying sorry." It feels like life or death, throwing them into survival mode, where they are more likely to become angry, shut down, deny, or become defensive. This is not because they don't care; it's because they care so much, and are now overwhelmed.

By showing our loyal and consistent warmth and safety, reminding them that mistakes are a normal part of being human, not a threat to who they are, we can help students overcome this sensitivity. Other students can benefit from learning not to take it personally if they don't get the apology they deserve because some people are extra sensitive to doing the right thing and apologising after doing the wrong thing. We can compassionately give each other time to develop the skill and highlight again, the importance of giving ourselves permission to be human.

Emphasise the importance of being accountable for actions and showing friends that you care enough to work through uncomfortable feelings of accountability, and to learn to apologise to mend friendship hurts. Encourage them to find other ways to show they are sorry, while they gather the courage to apologise.

Students who are particularly sensitive about saying sorry may experience a tight chest, a hot face, watery eyes, and an urge to become defensive, deny what happened, storm off, or release anger on the person. This happens because their brain is trying to protect them. It's worrying that if they did something wrong, people might be upset with them and no longer want to be friends. Their feelings about being liked and accepted can feel super strong inside. Their brain thinks, "Danger! I might lose someone I care about!" We know the truth is that making a mistake does not mean you will lose love or friendship.

Key takeaways from Chapter 7

- Conflict is a normal part of every friendship. Learning to handle it with courage and kindness helps friendships grow even stronger.
- Mistakes are opportunities! When you take responsibility, show empathy, and work to make things right, you build real trust.
- Empathy and perspective-taking are superpowers. They help you understand others, solve problems, and create lasting friendships.
- Positive actions, like listening, apologising, and communicating kindly, are the "glue" that hold friendships together. Hurtful actions, like leaving people out or being mean, can act as "erasers" and weaken those bonds.
- Healthy friendships need clear boundaries, honesty, and respect. It's important to notice not just what you meant, but how your actions made others feel.
- When you show you care, by listening, apologising, and trying to fix mistakes, you make your friendship (and your classroom!) a happier, safer place for everyone.
- Remember: Every day is a new chance to be a friendship hero. Small actions can make a big difference!

Call to action

Your friendship challenge: Ready to make a difference?

Every day is a new chance to be a friendship champion!. When things get tough, remember: every problem is a chance to learn, grow, and become a better friend. Use empathy, take responsibility, and speak up honestly and kindly. Whether you're helping to fix a friendship or supporting someone else, you're making your school and the world a kinder, happier place. Are you ready to take on the challenge and become a true friendship hero?

Let's normalise conflict as a learning opportunity (CASEL, 2020). Encourage empathy, responsibility, and respectful communication, so students build the skills and confidence for strong, supportive relationships.

References

Collaborative for Academic, Social, and Emotional Learning (CASEL). (2020). What is SEL? https://casel.org/what-is-sel/

Durlak, J. A., Weissberg, R. P., Dymnicki, A. B., Taylor, R. D., & Schellinger, K. B. (2011). The impact of enhancing students' social and emotional learning: A meta-analysis of school-based universal interventions. *Child Development*, 82(1), 405–432.

Goleman, D. (1995). *Emotional intelligence*. Bantam Books.

Hymel, S., Schonert-Reichl, K. A., & Miller, L. D. (2018). Social and emotional learning in schools: A Canadian perspective. In J. A. Durlak, C. E. Domitrovich, & J. L. Mahoney (Eds.), *Handbook of social and emotional learning* (pp. 407–424). Guilford Press.

Primrose, T. (2025, September 2). What is bullying. Keep Your Child Safe.org. https://keepyourchildsafe.org/bullying/learn-about-bullying/what-is-bullying/

Ruwa, R. (2025, August). *Can ADHD cause rejection sensitivity?* Healthline; Healthline Media. https://www.healthline.com/health/adhd-and-rejectionsensitivity

Appendix: Activities and ideas for friendship success

The following activities, games, and reflection prompts are designed to help students practise their friendship skills in fun and meaningful ways. Educators can use these directly or adapt them to suit their class. Students are also invited to contribute their own ideas and tips for building strong, positive friendships.

1. **Friendship scenarios role play**

   Choose a scenario (such as a misunderstanding at recess, a forgotten invitation, or sharing equipment). In groups or pairs, students act out both the problem and a positive solution, then discuss how it felt and what could be learned.

2. **Friendship Bingo**

   Create a Bingo board with boxes such as "Include someone new," "Apologise sincerely," "Help a friend in need," "Share something," "Listen carefully," etc. Students aim to complete a line or the whole card over a week.

3. **Compliment chain**

   Sit in a circle. One student gives a genuine compliment to another, who then passes it on to someone new. Continue until everyone has given and received a compliment. Reflect on how it feels to be kind and appreciated.

4. **Reflection prompts**
   - What was one thing you did this week that helped a friendship?
   - When did you use empathy or kindness to solve a problem?
   - How did it feel to apologise or forgive?
   - What can you do next time a conflict comes up?
5. **Friendship tips wall**

   Set up a space (physical or digital) where students can post their own advice for being a good friend. Encourage everyone to add their "top tip" or something that has worked for them.
6. **Student-created games**

   Challenge students to invent a new game or activity that encourages teamwork, kindness, or problem-solving. Play as a class and vote on your favourites.
7. **Friendship journals**

   Invite students to keep a journal where they record acts of kindness, challenges they faced in friendships, and what they learned each week.

Invite students to share new activities, games, or reflections for future editions of this appendix. Their creativity and experiences can help others on their own friendship quests!

Being yourself in friendships: Authenticity matters

When friendships are emotionally safe, genuine authenticity thrives, allowing friendships to develop honestly and comfortably, with the very best chance of lasting the test of time.

The learning quest: Embark on an adventure in self-discovery (Self-Awareness)

Imagine setting off on a quest where you are the hero! Throughout this adventure, you'll unlock your unique strengths, interests, and values, discovering treasures that only you possess. Instead of hiding or copying others to fit in, you'll gain powers of confidence, energy, and joy by embracing your authentic self. Along the way, exciting activities will help you express yourself boldly, set healthy boundaries, and celebrate what makes everyone different. Remember: true belonging is like joining a legendary team where everyone is valued for who they really are! When you stay true to yourself, you build friendships that last and create a world full of vibrant diversity and connection.

Trying to fit in by copying others or hiding who we are may help us get "accepted," but it drains energy, confidence, and joy. Authenticity means feeling like yourself, not changing to gain approval. Students reflect on their strengths, interests, and values, learning that self-acceptance fosters genuine connection. Activities guide students in expressing themselves, setting boundaries, and respecting others' individuality. True belonging is being accepted for who you are, while fitting in means changing who you are to

DOI: 10.4324/9781003617570-8

be accepted by others (Brown, 2010). Remaining true to ourselves creates genuine, lasting friendships and maintains social diversity (Brown, 2012).

Setting the scene (Chapter overview) (Self-Awareness, Communication Skills)

Searching for a sense of belonging and identity within a social group is a high priority during childhood and adolescence. While family can provide a steady foundation to step out from and safely back into, the social world is where our strengths and social–emotional intelligence are applied through conversation and play with people who won't automatically love and accept us the way family might. The social world has many moving parts, and the process of finding your place without compromising your authenticity and identity is uncomfortable and taxing for most young people.

Sometimes, children get lost in the noise and competition to fit in. Dominant personalities can emerge as everyone competes for social status. Those who need more time to develop self-awareness and confidence may end up in groups that don't reflect their true values. Instead, they may fit in by moulding themselves to group norms or hiding behind others' social positions. In doing so, they can lose touch with their own identity.

Social confidence starts with self-awareness, self-acceptance, and knowing your worth. It grows from genuine engagement and positive friendships, even if building it takes time and courage.

Strengths such as warmth, empathy, kindness, and honesty foster harmony more than academic or athletic success (Payton et al., 2000). Celebrating these soft skills builds deeper connections and well-being.

Confidence in your authentic self-thrives in cultures of compassion, equity, and psychological safety (Edmondson, 2019). These environments nurture well-being and genuine connections.

Open communication and trust help resolve conflict respectfully. Accountability and apologies come naturally, without affecting anyone's sense of belonging.

Balanced self-assurance allows us to approach friendships with kindness and respect without changing ourselves for others. This confidence relieves social pressure, making it easier to be authentic and to find supportive friends.

Being true to yourself—while respecting others and social norms—strengthens cultures of connection and belonging. Compassion and kindness help maintain psychological safety and well-being.

This chapter provides educators with strategies to help students be themselves, build confidence, and foster genuine friendships within an inclusive school culture.

Spotting the skills in action (Observation & Reflection) (Self-Awareness, Empathy, and Perspective Taking)

Share this case study with your students.

Leo's big idea

Leo loved planes. Real planes. Not the paper ones his class folded in art. He loved motors, wires, and circuits that sparked when he fixed them, but at school, none of that mattered. Everyone else loved football, basketball, and video games.

Leo tried to join in, but felt awkward and out of place. Pretending was exhausting.

Then there was Jasper. Jasper was always alone. Kids whispered about him or laughed when he walked by. He loved the same things Leo did: planes, gadgets, circuits, flying things. Leo had always liked Jasper, but was scared. "If I hang out with him, maybe the others will tease me too," Leo thought. One rainy Thursday, everyone ran inside. Leo sat on the bench, fiddling with a tiny motor. Sparks jumped when he tried to get it spinning.

"Hey," a voice said. Leo looked up. Jasper stood there, holding a small drone. "Want to help me test it?" Leo froze. His stomach knotted. The other kids would see. But the drone hummed like a song he couldn't ignore. "Okay," he whispered.

They crouched on the wet grass. Jasper smiled. "Try twisting the red wire." The drone spun and lifted. Leo gasped, "It worked!"

"See?" Jasper grinned. "Told you. You're good at this. "You too," Leo said, laughing. The first real laugh he'd had all week.

At lunch, Leo showed Jasper how a paper plane could fly. Some classmates stared, but Leo felt proud for being himself.

Soon, a couple of classmates wandered over, curious about what they were doing. They asked questions. Leo explained, Jasper added cool details, and before long, the soccer boys and basketball girls tried flying the paper planes too. Leo realised bravery wasn't kicking a ball far or pretending to know video games. Bravery was being himself, even when it scared him. And kindness? That was sharing what you loved with someone else, even if everyone else laughed.

By week's end, Leo felt lighter, lifted by joy and freedom from being himself.

Being himself was freeing. Leo realised, "Bravery is letting your true self soar."

Educator reflection

Do you feel your classroom has a strong foundation of psychological safety?

What have you noticed about the students who are most comfortable in their skin? Is there something about their character or mindset that helps?

What ideas have you used to help children like and express their genuine selves more?

How do you know a student isn't comfortable being themselves?

Do you remember what it was like to be the age your students are now? Do you remember being authentic and true to yourself back then?

Student reflection

Think about a part of the case study that reminds you of yourself or someone you know.

What did you learn from the story that could help if you or a friend ever feels like Leo?

Do you think your peers feel safe to be themselves around you?

Do you feel safe to be yourself around your friends?

Is there something about your answers that would be helpful to tell your teacher after this lesson, to help make your school culture stronger and happier?

Understanding the challenge of being yourself when fitting in matters so much. (Self-Awareness)

Being yourself feels great—unless your authenticity is rejected. Fitting in and social comparison are natural parts of growing up, and being yourself isn't always easy.

Invite students to close their eyes and reflect on their authenticity in class. With eyes closed, have them rate (0–10) how much they feel like themselves. Record responses anonymously and graph the results to show how comfortable students feel being themselves.

This exercise helps you support students in finding a sense of belonging and increases everyone's self-awareness, empathy, and compassion.

If you have an appropriate personal story about fitting in or being authentic, share it. Students value seeing vulnerability in adults.

Authenticity compliments circle

Building communities where everyone feels valued is everyone's responsibility. Open expression and diverse strengths fuel innovation and creativity (Armstrong, 2010; Edmondson, 2019). Authentic self-expression creates positive change and genuine friendships.

Seat students in a circle. Ask them to imagine what it feels like to pretend to be someone else to belong.

Look at each student, say their name, and share a unique character trait you admire. Then, have students in small groups find and share unique traits about each other.

Student reflection

How did it feel to receive a compliment about one of your character traits?

How did it feel to give a compliment about someone else's character?

What have you learned about the importance of being the kind of person people can be themselves around?

Blend or shine game (Self-Awareness, Communication Skills)

This game has two modes: moving together and moving differently.

Choose how you move or stay still—any style is welcome.

Movement ideas: stand, sit, kneel, gesture, sway, or rock—whatever feels comfortable.

The most important movement rule is to move in ways that keep our bodies and others' bodies safe.

Prepare two hand gestures to show blend mode and shine mode.

Time to begin

Begin in blend mode: show the gesture and say, "Copy my movement, big or small." Keep it slow and rhythmic.

Switch to shine mode: gesture and say, "Choose your own movement or stillness. There's no right or wrong."

Ideas include hand motions, rocking, swaying, stimming-friendly movements, quiet showing, and not performance.

Switch between modes every 20–30 seconds, using hand gestures each time.

Cool down transition

Return to stillness, place a hand on your chest or stomach, and take a slow breath together.

Student reflection

As you close this lesson, remind your students, "Belonging isn't about being the same.

Belonging is when everyone is safe to be themselves, and we help create that safety for each other." End with the question, "What could you do differently today, so that everyone feels safe to be their true self around you?"

Why being authentic matters for our friendships and ourselves. (Self-Awareness, Communication skills)

Discuss with students why it's important for people to feel safe being themselves. Use prompts to encourage reflection on authenticity.

It's easier to find the right friends and feel comfortable when you're authentic. Peers sense when you're pretending, so being yourself helps you connect.

People feel safer and trust genuine friends. If your group pressures you to act against your values, seek support and kinder friends. Being brave now saves future sadness.

Use your strengths to be yourself, and let others use theirs.

Your unique strengths shape who you are. Pretending exhausts you and keeps you from growing and finding the right friends. Pursuing people who don't value you damages confidence and well-being.

You'll feel happier and more relaxed when you stop trying to be someone else. If friends leave you anxious and exhausted, they may not be the right fit for you.

Building a school culture of authenticity. (Self-Awareness, Communication Skills, Empathy, and Perspective Taking)

School communities thrive when students, educators, and parents practice kindness, empathy, equity, and authenticity. Consistent, visible role modelling matters.

Remind students that actions create culture. Demonstrating kindness, compassion, and equity builds psychological safety and belonging.

The lift others up and be yourself movement

The Friendship Blueprint is a whole-school culture program that, when followed correctly, ensures all classes follow the same lessons each week, consistently enhancing school culture.

Arrange a whole-school meet-up. Invite a student leader or educator to briefly explain the purpose.

We're here to explore something important for every person standing here today. Psychological safety and authenticity, where everyone can be themselves and help others be themselves too. Psychological safety means feeling so comfortable and supported that you can share your ideas, feelings, and mistakes without being scared. Equity means everyone gets what they need to learn, grow, and shine, just like different plants need different amounts of sun and water. When we welcome diversity and let people be their true selves, our classroom and community become smarter, kinder, and more creative, because every person brings a special way of seeing and solving the world.

We're going to play a game where we get to feel what it's like to first blend in, secondly be ourselves, and lastly support each other as we all be ourselves.

When I call out "blend in," try to fit in with what people around you are doing. (This will require some volunteers to make sure enough students and teachers are actually doing something to blend in with). Look around, copy others, try to match them. Notice how your body feels while you're doing it. When I say freeze, freeze.

Next, I will call out, "Be yourself!" This is the authenticity zone. Here, you move in the way that feels most like the real you. You don't have to be loud. You don't have to impress. You just must be you. Big, small, silly, calm, focused, smooth, gentle, it all counts.

Lastly, I will call out "support each other!" This time, everyone keeps doing their thing, their way, but you support them by smiling, giving them a thumbs-up, and being kind to each other.

Now the instructions are clear, get ready to start the game. At the end of each section zone, invite students to reflect on how their body and mind felt after:

Blend in zone: "Check in with your body. Did that feel easy or hard? Was your breathing relaxed or tight? Did you feel like yourself or smaller?"
Authenticity zone: How did that feel inside? Being yourself feels different. It feels lighter. Braver. More like home.
Support zone: How did it feel to encourage others? How did it feel to be encouraged?

Closing statement from the principal.

When we try to **blend in**, everyone else seems to shrink.
When we are **authentic**, everyone gets braver.
And when we **support one another**, our school becomes a safer place for everyone.
Your real self is a gift to this community. And so is everyone else's.
Students return to class together.

> **Educator reflection**
> Authenticity can look quiet, still, subtle, or minimal. All are valid. How do you think your students did with this activity? Would you do it again? If so, what would you change to improve it?

> **Student reflection**
> Where is one place you can try to be yourself more this week?
> Who are five children and/or adults you can be yourself with?
> If you don't feel psychologically safe at school, who could help you?

Finding your authentic and genuine strengths. (Self-Awareness, Empathy, and Perspective Taking)

"Be yourself, everyone else is taken." (author unknown).
Discussion and role plays

Write this quote on the board and invite your students to discuss it. Remind them that with strengths come weaknesses, and together, we can lift each other up and fill in each other's gaps. Encourage students to embrace their unique gifts rather than following trends or trying to be someone they're not.

Role Plays. (Self-Awareness, Communication Skills, Conflict Resolution, and Problem Solving)

The following role plays give children and adolescents an opportunity to explore different responses to the pressure to fit in or be authentic within a friendship group. Each scenario challenges them to consider their values, self-worth, and the consequences of their actions. By allowing them to navigate these situations, they can develop the confidence and skills necessary to stand up for their authenticity and cultivate healthy, genuine friendships.

The role plays provide them with a framework to practice identifying when a friendship is no longer aligned with their core values. Students can experiment with different approaches to navigating difficult situations, such as having honest conversations, gradually distancing themselves, or taking the risk of moving on from a friendship. By practising these scenarios, children can learn how to honour themselves and their values, while also fostering respectful and supportive relationships.

Role Play 1: Style pressure

All your friends dress similarly. You've been feeling pressure to dress the same way to fit in, even though it's not really your style.
Your choices.

1. Buy an outfit like theirs and wear it, even if it's not your style.
   Outcome: You wear the outfit, but you feel uncomfortable all day. You realise that trying to be someone else isn't making you happy. Later, you decide to talk to your friends about how much you enjoy your unique style, and they turn out to be supportive.
2. Wear something you feel comfortable in and own it confidently.
   Outcome: Some friends might comment on your outfit, but you stay true to yourself. By the end of the day, your friends respect your choice and even start complimenting you on your individuality. They appreciate you for being authentic.
3. Avoid dressing like your friends and distance yourself from the group.
   Outcome: You start to feel isolated because the group isn't connecting with you as much. You realise that it's important to have friends who respect your true self. You have a heart-to-heart conversation with your group, explaining why it's important for you to be authentic, and they begin to understand.

Role Play 2: The secret you can't keep

You've found out something about one of your friends that could potentially hurt the group, and you're unsure whether you should tell anyone or keep it a secret.

Your choices.

1. Keep the secret and hope the situation resolves itself.
   Outcome: You feel guilty and stressed because keeping the secret doesn't sit well with you. The situation escalates, and you end up feeling alienated because you didn't speak up. Later, you learn the importance of being honest and helping your friends when they need it.
2. Discuss the secret with the friend who shared it and encourage them to share it with the group if necessary.
   Outcome: Your friend feels supported by you and eventually opens up to the group. The conversation is tough, but everyone learns the importance of honesty. You feel proud of helping your friend and being true to your values.
3. Share the secret with the group, thinking it might help.
   Outcome: The group reacts strongly, leading to tension. Some friends might be upset with you for not respecting privacy. You realise that while honesty is important, respecting boundaries and finding the right way to address concerns is key.

Role Play 3: "Everyone's doing it" pressure

Your friends want you to be part of something you're uncomfortable with, like making fun of another person or gossiping about someone. You feel torn between wanting to fit in and not wanting to hurt someone else.

Your choices.

1. Go along with it, hoping you can avoid feeling guilty later.
   Outcome: You participate in the gossip, but later feel ashamed and regret your actions. You realise that true friends will respect you for standing up for what's right, and you vow not to let peer pressure change your values again.
2. Speak up and tell your friends you don't feel comfortable doing it.
   Outcome: Some friends might be disappointed or surprised, but they respect your decision. Over time, they come to understand the

importance of kindness, and your relationship grows stronger because of your honesty and integrity.

3. Temporarily distance yourself from the group and reflect on what truly matters to you.
   Outcome: You take some time to think about your boundaries and values. When you talk to your friends again, let them know that you don't want to engage in hurtful behaviour. Your friends may feel awkward at first, but they will eventually begin to respect your decision, and you will develop more meaningful friendships.

Role Play 4: The gossip group

You've been part of a friendship group where everyone often talks negatively about others behind their backs. You've been feeling uncomfortable because it goes against your values of kindness and respect.
   Your choices.

1. Speak up and express how uncomfortable you feel with the gossip.
   Outcome: You tell the group, "I don't feel good about talking negatively about others. I believe we should lift people up instead of bringing them down." Some friends may not understand, but a couple of them agree with you. Over time, the group either respects your viewpoint or drifts apart from it.
2. Gradually distance yourself from the group.
   Outcome: You start spending more time with friends who share your values. You no longer engage in the gossip sessions. While the group may start to feel distant, you feel relieved, knowing you're staying true to yourself. Ultimately, the friendships that remain are healthier and more aligned with your values.
3. Ignore your discomfort and keep gossiping.
   Outcome: You go along with the gossip, but the discomfort grows. Eventually, you realise that continuing to fit in with the group is making you feel worse. This teaches you that compromising your values for the sake of friendship isn't worth it in the long run.

Role Play 5: Peer pressure

You've been hanging out with a group that encourages risky or mean behaviour, like excluding others or breaking rules, which goes against your sense of fairness and kindness.

Your choices.

1. Express your discomfort with the behaviour and suggest an alternative way to act.
   Outcome: You say, "I don't think it's right to exclude others or break the rules. I think we should be kind to everyone." Some friends might get upset, but others agree with you. The group either shifts its behaviour, or you naturally grow apart from friends who don't share your values.
2. Stop hanging out with the group and find others who share your values.
   Outcome: You begin to distance yourself from the group, and although it's hard at first, you start finding friends who treat others with respect and kindness. You feel a sense of relief and peace because you no longer feel pressured to act against your values.
3. Stay in the group but feel conflicted inside.
   Outcome: You continue to participate in the behaviour to fit in, but the internal conflict intensifies. Eventually, you reach a point where you can't continue, and you make the decision to walk away from the group, knowing that it was the right choice for your peace of mind.

Role Play 6: The group's judgment

You're in a group where everyone judges others based on things like appearance, social status, or popularity. This makes you feel uncomfortable because you value kindness and acceptance, even when they are absent.

Your choices.

1. Stand up for inclusion and express that judgment isn't okay.
   Outcome: You say, "I don't think it's fair to judge people based on looks or status. We should accept people for who they are." Some friends may not understand, but others start to think about how they treat others. In time, the group may either change or grow apart.
2. Start distancing yourself from the group and spending more time with like-minded friends.
   Outcome: You stop hanging out with the group as much and find friends who value inclusivity and kindness. You start feeling more comfortable

and confident in your new friendships, knowing that you're aligning with people who share your values.

3. Pretend to go along with the group and suppress your discomfort.
   Outcome: You continue to feel conflicted, as the judgment weighs on you. Over time, you realise that pretending isn't worth it, and you decide to have an honest conversation about your values and how you can't participate in that kind of behaviour anymore.

Role Play 7 "Fake" friend

One of your close friends has started to act insincerely towards you. They're constantly pretending to be something they're not, which makes you feel uncomfortable because you value honesty and authenticity.
  Your choices.

1. Discuss your feelings with your friend.
   Outcome: You say, "I feel like you're not being yourself around me. I truly value honesty and authenticity. I wish you would be more authentic with me." Your friend might not understand, but you've expressed your feelings. If the behaviour continues, you decide to step away from the friendship gradually.
2. Gradually distance yourself from this friend.
   Outcome: You start distancing yourself from the friend and spending more time with people who are more authentic. Eventually, you realise that this friend's actions no longer align with your values, and you choose to move on to healthier friendships.
3. Ignore the behaviour and continue being friends.
   Outcome: You ignore your feelings and continue pretending to be okay with the situation. Over time, you begin to feel drained and unhappy. Eventually, you realise that holding onto this friendship isn't worth sacrificing your values, and you decide to part ways.

Role Play 8 Different priorities

You and your friends have very different priorities. They spend most of their time on social media and focusing on popularity, while you prefer nature walks with friends and family, kicking the football around, and helping others. The difference in priorities is causing tension.

Your choices:

1. Explain your values and priorities to your friends.
   Outcome: You tell your friends, "I really like it when we go out walking together and chatting. I feel like I'm not connecting with you as much when we focus so much on social media." Some friends might not understand, but a few will respect your priorities. You eventually find people with similar values and grow closer to them.
2. Start spending more time with people who share your interests.
   Outcome: You gradually spend less time with your current friends and engage in activities that align with your values. You make new friends who appreciate your interests, and the change feels empowering and positive.
3. Pretend to share your friends' priorities.
   Outcome: You try to fit in by pretending to enjoy social media and focusing on popularity, but it leaves you feeling unfulfilled. Eventually, you realise that staying true to your own values is far more important than trying to fit into a group where you no longer feel authentic.

Educator reflection

What more do you think your students need to understand to help increase psychological safety in your class, so everyone feels safe being kind, equitable, and authentic?

Diverse communities are stronger communities. (Empathy and Perspective Taking, Communication Skills)

Growing up in 1980s Australia, I saw children singled out for being different, by culture, ability, or appearance. This taught me how crucial it is to value diversity and create communities where everyone feels included. Personally, I experienced isolation and exclusion that was openly connected to my cultural heritage. Later in high school, the low-hanging fruit was my skin colour, and the same taunting happened to peers based on their skin, hair, size, or height, focus on study or lack thereof. I wasn't the only one, and it wasn't as personal as it seems these days. Being teased about your colour or height is something that you don't work hard for or earn. They are inherited genetic predispositions that just happen. I really don't know why people give so much weight to someone's value based on their height or perceived beauty, given they didn't have to work on either, and neither has anything to do with a person's worth or ability to contribute positively to society.

Today, bullying seems much more personal, and the taunts are far cleverer and more personal, cutting much deeper than what I experienced.

I hope this chapter will help strengthen our communities by enabling all young people to understand and appreciate the wonderfully diverse ways humans inhabit the earth and to leave behind discrimination and inequity.

Understanding neurodivergence

In my survey of young people around Australia, over 50% of children didn't know what neurodivergent meant. Here is one definition, and of course, feel free to find one that resonates with you:

> Neurodivergent describes people whose brains are significantly different from what is expected in the 'typical' population. That means they have different strengths and challenges compared to people whose brains don't exhibit those differences. The possible differences might be innate (e.g., Autism) or acquired (e.g., brain injury) and include medical conditions (e.g., epilepsy), mental health conditions (e.g., trauma), learning disabilities (e.g., dyslexia), and other neurodevelopmental conditions (e.g., ADHD).
>
> (Armstrong, 2010; Silberman, 2015).
> (Dr Melanie Heyworth, Founder and Head
> of Research at 'Reframing Autism')

Explaining to your students that neurodivergence is a term used to describe brains that have different strengths and challenges from those of people whose brains don't exhibit these differences is a helpful starting point.

From there, we want all young people to understand one more term to open their hearts and minds to a happier, more connected, neuroaffirming world. This is all about being the kind of person who prioritises the dignity and worth of all people, regardless of their cognitive differences.

For schools and communities to have the best chance of coexisting and growing together through everyone's unique and valuable presence, we need cultures that celebrate the strengths and advantages of all brains every day, not just on publicised "awareness days."

Different brains have different strengths, mini clips

Invite your students to create short video clips to send home to their parents and present to the class on what neurodivergence and neuroaffirming mean to them. Using age-appropriate explanations like, "Everyone's brain works in a unique way, and every person can use their brain's strengths to support a better life for them and for the world. Some people are skilled at noticing small details, while others excel at thinking creatively. Some brains don't pick up social cues the same way others do, but they still care about their friends. All these brains are strong, healthy, and valuable."

Experiencing the wonder and awe of our different brains, a short conversation

Show your excitement about how much you've learnt and grown over the years, as you met hundreds of wonderfully rich and unique brains to teach over the years. Share a story about how many times, as a child, you felt and saw other children feel confused when something unexpected happened during playtime, and that you now understand this was probably a situation where your brain's strengths and thinking style were different from the other child's strengths and thinking style. If you don't understand neurodivergence, you might simply brush off people with different thinking, communication, and cultural styles, thinking maybe you're too different to become friends.

From quick judgment to thoughtful reflection and compassion, when a social situation feels puzzling

Often, children don't know what to think or say when navigating a neuro-divergent friend, and a social mishap occurs. Talk to your students about the kinds of situations they might have experienced where their intuition told them the person's intent didn't match the impact. Validate mixed feelings while teaching empathy. It's natural for your students to feel confused, hurt, or even annoyed when a student unintentionally upsets them, and the impact has been profound. Acknowledge their feelings if they are unhappy after a social mishap with words like: "It makes sense that you felt upset. Let's think about why they might have acted that way." There is always a way to guide them toward empathy without invalidating their experience.

Offer the following ideas for thinking and communicating through one of these moments and share how this increases their compassion and empathy, which in turn improves their own and the other person's social-emotional well-being.

Questions students can ask themselves when observing a social mishap:
"I wonder if they meant that differently?"
"Could they be nervous, shy, or thinking differently about this?"
"What else could be going on for this person?"
"If they didn't mean to hurt someone, how could we help them understand?"
"Maybe they didn't know."
"Let's help each other understand."
"Could I explain things differently to them?"
"Instead of thinking 'that was rude,' you can ask yourself, 'Did they know that might hurt someone's feelings?'"

Friendly, supportive language they can use to help their friend understand a social misstep
"Hey, just so you know, that might have sounded a bit harsh. Do you want to try saying it another way?"
"I don't think they liked that. Want me to help you figure out what happened?"
"I know you didn't mean to hurt anyone. Let's fix it together."

Role plays to practice compassionate, non-judgmental communication

Allow some time for your students to work together in pairs or small groups to role-play the concepts discussed and develop compassionate communication tools to support each other during social mishaps without judgment or criticism.

Neurodivergence film clips

Return to the definitions of neurodivergence and neuroaffirming. Provide students with an opportunity to film short clips sharing their personal perspectives and understandings, along with one way they know neurodivergence helps advance the world. Share the clips with parents, carers, and other classes to support everyone's growth through diverse thinking and perspectives across the community. Include your own clip too.

Our shared humanity and cultures of friendship from around the world (Empathy and Perspective Taking, Communication Skills)

When we don't see eye to eye with someone, frustration is natural. Compassion, empathy, and kindness take practice and are easier in cultures that support them (Gilbert, 2009).

One of the ways I've found easiest, both as a professional working with young people and as a parent, to be less reactive and more compassionate is to remember our shared humanity. A day does not go by that my first morning thoughts are not those that remind me I'm just like everyone else. We all wake up wanting to have a great day. No one wants to experience emotional discomfort and pain. By starting my day with a wish for all beings to be happy and well, I can meet the day with an open heart, patience, and compassion, whenever I feel myself heat up with stress and overwhelm. It doesn't get me through every tough moment, but it helps me remain kind and compassionate in all circumstances. My day begins with the question, "How do I want to be today?" and ends with "What do I want to do better tomorrow?"

We're all connected by our shared humanity. Our brains are wired for survival, not happiness, making us all vulnerable to stress and anxiety (Siegel, 2012).

We all suffer, we all have joy, we all strive, we all rise, and sometimes fall. The human experience is both vastly different and yet remarkably similar. Connecting deeply with our shared humanity reminds us that we all want the best for ourselves, everyone makes mistakes, and we all learn at our own pace. If we want others to be understanding with us, we need to be understanding of others.

If we want connected communities, we need to learn from one another and grow in as many ways as possible, enriching our own lives and those of others, making them richer and happier.

Learning from other cultures

Friendship, connection, and belonging are valued in all cultures. No matter where you look in the world, social groups are sought after and valued. As a Sri Lankan-born Australian, I have loved learning from both cultures and the different ways friendships are enhanced and celebrated. In Sri Lanka, friendship is often demonstrated through acts of service and generosity, rooted in empathy and compassion for one another. Even people with few resources and poor health will generously do what they can to uplift and support their fellow humans. For years, I watched my parents, new migrants who left everything behind in Sri Lanka to give their young children new opportunities, never complain about what they had lost and left behind, and instead, reach out to fellow University students and help so many of them as they too, adjusted to their new lives here in Australia. I saw it again as a 10-year-old when my beautiful Dad passed away suddenly from a short illness. Mum, always kind, stoic, honest, and generous, didn't get stuck in her own sorrow (and there was plenty of that, losing the love of her life at just 42), but she put that energy into making things better for her friends and for my dad's friends. She cooked, she cared, and she kept her regular visits to elderly Sri Lankans as part of her routine. I see that my family and friends continue to do the same. Always ready to help, always happy to host, and generous with their presence and service with no expectation of return. I saw in Australia how friendships were strengthened through conversation, shared hobbies and interests, humour, light-hearted, playful teasing, sharing food, and gathering to watch sports. I know that both cultures have much more to them, and how they celebrate and honour friendship, but these are my strongest memories and experiences.

Take a moment to share with your students what friendship culture you've been exposed to, and then invite them to share any of their experiences.

Next, enthusiastically share the joyful meanings behind the word "friendship" in the following cultures and open a discussion about what we can learn from and apply in our own lives.

Ubuntu *(Zulu/Southern Africa)* "I am because we are."
A philosophy expressing shared humanity, compassion, and the interconnectedness of all people. Friendship is belonging to one another and the value of *community before self.*

Kalyana Mitra *(Sinhala/Sri Lankan Buddhist tradition)* "Virtuous friend."
Refers to a friend who uplifts, guides, and supports one's moral and spiritual growth. Sri Lankans will rarely be heard saying they can't help when asked for support. Acts of service are among the most valued ways they show support and friendship.

Ceol agus craic *(Irish)*
Meaning music and good fun. Friends come together to sing, tell stories, and celebrate life. Giving someone a Claddagh ring is a special way to symbolise love, loyalty, and friendship, and is also a traditional Irish gesture of connection.

Nakama *(Japanese)* "Close companion or kindred spirit."
Describes deep friendships where people share common goals and mutual trust, like family.

Amistad *(Spanish)* "Friendship."
Rooted in warmth, loyalty, and genuine affection between people.

Dosti *(Hindi/India)* "Friendship."
A cherished bond of loyalty, laughter, and support often considered sacred and lifelong.

Whanaungatanga *(Māori/New Zealand)* "Kinship, sense of family connection."
A concept extending beyond family ties. This is about friendship, belonging, and shared experiences that unite people.

Camaraderie *(French)* "Mutual trust and cheerful friendship."
Friendship forged through shared experiences, often among colleagues or teammates.

Sobremesa *(Spanish-speaking cultures)* "Over the table."
The warmth and connection shared after a meal when friends linger to talk. Friendship through togetherness.

Philia *(Ancient Greek)* "Affectionate regard or deep friendship."
One of the highest forms of love in Greek philosophy, showing loyalty and virtuousness, based on mutual respect.
Amitié *(French)* "Friendship."
Expresses affection, kindness, and the joy of companionship, often associated with trust and emotional closeness.

Across the world, friendships may take different forms; through gifts, food, time, or words, but the message remains the same: friends show care, respect, and loyalty in ways that make each other feel valued and connected.

Divide your students into pairs and assign them a culture from the previous list, or have them conduct their own research or draw on their personal experiences.

In their assigned pairs (or small groups), invite them to choose a way to express their new understanding of how another culture celebrates friendship. Ideas include creating a poster, a short skit, a musical performance, artwork, or a Role-Play.

Allow time for your students to think deeply about the culture they are representing. Be sure to share their work with other classes through an exhibition, an assembly, or by exchanging it.

Neurodivergence and cultural friendship guide. (Empathy and Perspective Taking, Communication Skills)

As we come to the end of this chapter, students can create their own book about friendship, bringing together what they've learnt about neurodivergence and cultures from around the world. You might even consider contacting the local newspaper to share how you're helping connect communities through deep knowledge and compassion.

Allow students a couple of weeks to research. Younger students will require considerable support to accomplish this. Support students to create a title that reflects the area they studied, and answer as many of the following questions as possible. Consider binding your book, publishing it, and donating a copy to your local library, or selling copies for a school fundraiser.

Title

Facts about XYZ

Myths about XYZ

Strengths that I admire about XYZ

Friendship qualities that are common in XYZ

Some ways XYZ can be misunderstood in friendships.

The most interesting thing I learnt about XYZ

Character traits about XYZ that I share.

My Friendship Blueprint goal that shows I value XYZ and support their equity, inclusion, and belonging at our school:

Key takeaways. Make your learning legendary!

- Every friendship adventure begins with self-awareness, courage, and the superpower of being true to yourself. When you embrace your quirks and strengths, you attract friends who appreciate the real you!
- Belonging is like finding a team where you can wear your favourite colours and still be cheered on, no need to change who you are to fit in.
- Empathy, communication, and problem-solving are your magical tools for building strong, inclusive friendships and communities.
- Embracing all kinds of brains and learning about cultures from around the world turns your friendship quest into an epic, colourful journey, where everyone feels valued and included!
- Every act of kindness, authenticity, and support is like levelling up your friendship powers, making your relationships stronger and your classroom a happier place for all.

Your next move: Take the friendship challenge, a call to action

Are you ready to become a friendship hero? Use what you've learned to celebrate your uniqueness, lift others up, and lead by example! Stand up for kindness, include everyone, and encourage your friends to let their true colours shine. Start a chain reaction: make one bold, authentic choice today, and watch your classroom transform into a place where every friendship thrives. Remember, being yourself is the greatest gift you can give to your friends and your school!

References

Armstrong, T. (2010). *The power of neurodiversity: Unleashing the advantages of your differently wired brain*. Da Capo Lifelong.

Brown, B. (2010). *The gifts of imperfection: Let go of who you think you're supposed to be and embrace who you are*. Hazelden.

Brown, B. (2012). *Daring greatly: How the courage to be vulnerable transforms the way we live, love, parent, and lead*. Penguin Random House Audio Publishing Group.

Edmondson, A. C. (2019). *The fearless organization: Creating psychological safety in the workplace for learning, innovation, and growth*. John Wiley & Sons, Inc.

Gilbert, P. (2009). *The compassionate mind*. Constable and Robinson.

Miller, C. (2024, January 16). *Helping kids make friends - Child mind institute*. Child Mind Institute. https://childmind.org/give/newsletters/helping-kids-make-friends/

National Scientific Council on the Developing Child. (2015). *Supportive relationships and active skill-building strengthen the foundations of resilience*. (Working Paper No. 13). Center on the Developing Child at Harvard University. https://developingchild.harvard.edu/resources/working-paper/supportive-relationships-and-active-skill-building-strengthen-the-foundations-of-resilience/

Payton, J. W., Wardlaw, D. M., Graczyk, P. A., Bloodworth, M. R., Tompsett, C. J., & Weissberg, R. P. (2000). Social and emotional learning: A framework for promoting mental health and reducing risk behavior in children and youth. *Journal of School Health, 70*(5), 179–185.

Siegel, D. J. (2012). *The developing mind: How relationships and the brain interact to shape who we are* (2nd ed.). Guilford Press.

Silberman, S. (2015). *Neurotribes: the legacy of autism and the future of neurodiversity*. Avery.

Appendix: Bonus activities and resources to supercharge your friendship quest

Friendship quest journal prompts

- What makes you feel most like yourself?
- Write about a time you were brave enough to be authentic.
- List five strengths that make you a great friend.
- Draw your "Friendship Superhero" and their powers!

Games and energizers

- Compliment circle remix: Each student gives a compliment in a silly voice or with a fun gesture.
- "Find Your Match" scavenger hunt: Students find classmates who share unique interests or strengths.
- Secret kindness missions: Draw a secret mission card with a kind act to complete during the week.

Creative challenges

- Create a classroom mural celebrating what makes everyone unique.
- Write a rap, poem, or short story about an unforgettable friendship adventure.
- Design "Friendship Badges" to award for acts of kindness and authenticity.

Reflection and growth

- Weekly "Level Up" check-ins: How did you help a friend or show your true self this week?
- Friendship goal tracker: Set and track personal goals for being a supportive, inclusive friend.

Keep questing, keep growing, and let your true self shine!

Choosing the right friends and navigating social roadblocks

Choosing the right friends is important because when we're in safe and friendly company, we feel relaxed and ready to play and grow.

Learning quest: The adventure of friendship! (Self-Awareness)

Get ready for an epic quest. Imagine you're a Friendship Explorer on a mission to discover what makes a great friend and how to handle tricky social situations. Each lesson is a new adventure, think of it like a video game where you level up your friendship skills. The more you practice, the stronger your friendship powers become!

Social conflict is part of life, but children can learn to handle it while staying true to themselves (Bagwell & Schmidt, 2011; Rubin et al., 2015). This chapter teaches students how to avoid gossip, conflict spirals, and peer pressure and find friends who make them feel respected and safe (Olweus, 1993; Durlak et al., 2011). The "right friends" aren't perfect—they're those who let you be yourself.

This chapter provides strategies for handling social conflict and choosing real friends (Bukowski et al., 2018; Wentzel & Caldwell, 1997). Students will learn what makes friendships healthy, how friends affect behaviour and self-esteem (Rose & Rudolph, 2006), and how to handle peer pressure (Steinberg & Monahan, 2007). Through reflection, they'll develop their own criteria for positive friendships.

DOI: 10.4324/9781003617570-9

Setting the scene

Remember your first day at school or day care? Alone, surrounded by strangers, many of us just wanted someone to make us feel safe. From the beginning, belonging and purpose are what matter most.

Friendship is complex, especially as young people's brains are still developing and shaped by mood, hormones, and social pressures (Blakemore & Mills, 2014; Güroğlu, 2022b). My hope is that every child finishes this book knowing they deserve belonging, connection, and to feel their life matters.

Authentic, consistent friendships are crucial to self-esteem (Antonopoulou et al., 2019; Bagwell & Schmidt, 2011). While we can't control backgrounds, we can shape a positive social environment. Teaching prosocial friendship skills in schools can change lives for generations (Durlak et al., 2011).

Early friendships often form easily over shared interests. As children grow, their personalities and interests diversify, and relationships become more complex. These moments shape social confidence and well-being.

Belonging and peer connections shape our identity and sense of safety (Allen & Bowles, 2012). As we grow, friendships become more about shared values, empathy, and respect. Our need to belong can sometimes lead to poor choices, but we thrive together (Swedell, 2012; Waite, 2021).

Friends shape our well-being (Rubin et al., 2015). Young people should look for friends with similar values who let them be themselves. Kindness and respect help build a positive school culture (Durlak et al., 2011). We can always improve by adopting good habits and using our strengths.

This chapter encourages students to be the friend they need and seek those who help build a positive school culture—supporting through challenges, celebrating successes, offering kind feedback, and respecting boundaries and individuality.

Spotting the skills in action (Observation and Reflection) (Empathy and Perspective Taking, Self-Awareness)

Meet Marley! Marley is someone who loves to laugh, play fair, and make sure everyone feels included. But starting at a new school,

Marley quickly discovered that making friends isn't always easy. What would you do if you were Marley? Let's step into Marley's shoes and figure it out together!

At first, Marley found a group of school friends who seemed fun. They invited Marley to sit with them, whispering secrets and giggling. Marley felt lucky and relieved. Finally, a place to belong.

Even though Marley felt much better with his new friends than he ever felt being alone, something felt strange. The group had rules that were never spoken aloud, yet they were somehow expected. He had to laugh when they laughed (even if someone got hurt) and could only talk to certain people. His feelings didn't seem to matter to them as much as following their group rules. If he didn't follow these rules exactly, they would look at him funny, whisper and laugh, and sometimes even completely ignore him.

One day, the group's leader, Imogen, told Marley, "Don't sit with Tessa tomorrow. She said You're annoying." Marley felt a sting in their chest. Tessa? My friend? Marley didn't want to believe it, but Imogen said it so confidently, as if it were a fact.

The next day, Marley sat far away from Tessa. Later, Tessa came over to Marley, her eyes wide with confusion. "Why didn't you sit with me?" she asked softly. "I… heard you didn't like me anymore," Marley replied. Tessa shook her head. "I never said that. Who told you that?" Marley's heart tightened. Something is wrong.

The next week, Marley noticed: friends whispered secrets, then denied it; told Marley something, then blamed him for sharing; acted friendly one day, cold the next.

Marley felt lost in a maze of confusion, but the deepest pain was the loneliness that followed.

One afternoon, Marley found someone sitting alone in the music room. Their name was Jonah, and they looked happy and content, quietly drawing aeroplanes. Jonah looked up and smiled a small, real smile; the kind of smile that didn't ask anything from you. Marley sat down beside Jonah. They didn't talk at first. They didn't have to. After a while, Marley asked, "How do you know who your real friends are?" Jonah thought carefully and said, "Real friends make you feel like more of yourself, not less."

The words landed softly in Marley's chest, like puzzle pieces finally clicking. Marley realised something very important: True belonging isn't about fitting into any group; it's feeling secure enough to be your real self. Marley thought about those words all afternoon, and he slept well that night.

The next day, Marley did something brave, so brave it was terrifying. When Imogen tried to whisper another instruction, Marley stood tall and said, "No, thank you. I like choosing my own friends." There was silence. A tense, sticky silence. Right at that moment, Jonah waved from across the yard. Marley walked towards him, his heart steady, and his steps sure.

Over time, Marley made new friends and repaired things with Tessa, learning valuable lessons about true connection along the way.

Marley stopped searching for a big crowd or for the safety of hiding behind the tough, popular students. All he needed was a few kind friends who felt 'right' to be with. Marley's laughter soon returned, not because life was perfect, but because he was true to himself and his friends.

Student reflection

Why do you think Marley felt even lonelier with the new group of friends?

How do you know a friend wants the best for you?

If you could give one piece of advice to the unkind students to help them, see how important it is to rethink their behaviour, what would it be?

Educator reflection

How easy is it to tell if relational aggression is happening in your class?

How do you know social conflict is happening?

What do you think will help reduce social conflict right across the school?

What to look for in a friend. (Self-Awareness, Empathy, and Perspective Taking)

Sometimes, students choose friends to avoid loneliness, even if those friendships are unhealthy (Bagwell & Schmidt, 2011). Belonging is a basic need, but not all friendships are supportive (Rubin et al., 2015).

Every culture teaches that a good life starts with how we treat others. Differences in personality and emotion have caused conflict between friends, families, and countries for centuries.

Even knowing someone is a negative influence doesn't always make it easy to avoid them. People make unhealthy friendship choices for many reasons—fear, insecurity, loneliness, or low confidence.

The Friendship Blueprint teaches warmth, kindness, empathy, inclusion, respect, honesty, and authenticity (CASEL, 2020). Students need time to consolidate these skills as their brains mature.

We can best support students by encouraging kindness and helping them avoid relational aggression. Positive change takes time, and not all social cultures shift quickly, but every effort helps.

This lesson clarifies what is and isn't encouraged in school friendships. Share "The Friendship Blueprint do's and don'ts" poster to guide students (Figure 9.1).

The red, orange, and green light connection map

Hand out paper and markers, and let students reflect privately, away from others. Remind them not to share answers to maintain a safe atmosphere. Collect answers when finished and assure students their responses are confidential.

Give students time to consider which friends are uplifting, draining, or in between. If needed, do this activity one-on-one for added safety.

Creating the map

Students draw a circle to fill the page. They place themselves in the middle. Around this circle, they can draw the names of all their classmates.

Lines are drawn between them and each of their peers to represent how they feel within that connection.

Thick line = Green light. I feel safe with this person.

Thin line = Orange light. Sometimes I feel okay, sometimes I don't.

Dotted line = Red light. It feels uncomfortable and unsafe to be friends.

THE FRIENDSHIP BLUEPRINT

HOW TO BE AN AWESOME FRIEND!

Friendship challenges can be tough, but when everyone does their part, our school gets stronger and more welcoming for everyone!

DO'S:
HOW TO BUILD STRONG FRIENDSHIPS.

✓ Do — Be honest and trustworthy.

✓ Do — Be kind and friendly.

✓ Do — Make healthy choices for your body and mind.

✓ Do — Notice and care about others.

✓ Do — Be kind to your mind and others' minds too.

✓ Do — Respect boundaries and let people make their own choices.

DON'TS:
WHAT TO AVOID SO FRIENDSHIPS STAY STRONG.

✗ Don't — Gossip.

✗ Don't — Be mean on purpose.

✗ Don't — Use gossip or exclusion to hurt others.

✗ Don't — Lie.

✗ Don't — Exclude others.

✗ Don't — Blame others; take responsibility for your actions.

✗ Don't — Think everyone else is the problem—happy schools are a team effort. We all help!

✗ Don't — Use your feelings to hurt others on purpose.

Remind students not to share or compare answers. Emphasise empathy and confidentiality (Bauminger-Zviely, 2013). Watch out for neurodivergent students, who may be more vulnerable to peer manipulation.

Handle the connection map with care. Student responses can provide valuable insights and reveal patterns that need attention.

Students who are marked red or orange may be struggling more than they appear. Collect their work and move to the next activity.

Team echo

In this game, students will connect positively through sound and rhythm (while letting off steam from the more taxing content of the previous activity). Start by having a student or educator make a simple sound or rhythm (e.g., clap-clap, click-click, tap-tap, shake-shake).

The group **echoes** the sound back in their own way. They can match it exactly or choose a *gentle variation* that feels good (slower, quieter, different movement).

Let students take turns as sound leaders. Remind everyone to keep a safe tone. Provide headphones or space for those who need it.

If possible, end the lesson outside so students can move around and reconnect.

Boundaries. (Self-Awareness, Communication Skills, Conflict Resolution, and Problem Solving)

It's easy to forget how hard it is for young people to say "no" when everyone else is saying "yes," or to set boundaries when they long to belong.

Setting boundaries can feel risky for young people who are afraid of losing friends. Self-awareness helps them find the right friends and know when to step back from conflict. This lesson develops self-awareness through the idea of an inner compass.

Group brainstorm

Ask the group: "What kinds of things might cross a friend's boundary?"

Guide them to consider social, physical, emotional, and digital boundaries.

Examples might include:

Social: Excluding someone from a game, interrupting, not taking "no" for an answer.

Physical: Touching without permission, grabbing things, and standing too close.

Emotional: Teasing, name-calling, sharing secrets without permission.

Digital: Sending mean messages, posting photos without asking, tagging someone in something they don't like.

Record their ideas on the board under each category.

Scenario discussion

Present the boundary crossing scenarios that follow, and at the end of each one, ask:

> "Who do you think feels uncomfortable?"
> "What boundary might be crossed?"
> "What could the child say or do to set a boundary?"

Boundary-crossing social scenarios

A friend keeps taking your pencil even after you say, "Please don't."
Someone makes a joke about the way you look and laughs.
A friend posts a photo of you online without asking.
During a game, someone refuses to let you join.
A friend hugs you even though you said "no thanks."
Encourage multiple answers and validate all children's feelings.

> ### Reflection
> Ask: "Why is it important to set boundaries with friends?"

Highlight

Boundaries keep everyone safe and respected.
Friends who listen to boundaries build stronger friendships.

We all have the right to say what we are okay with, and good friends will respect that. It's okay to say: "Please stop, I don't like that." "That's not okay with me." "I need some space right now." "I don't want to be teased; it hurts my feelings." "Please don't talk to me like that." "I said no, and I mean it." "I don't want to share that right now." "That's my choice, and I'd like you to respect it." "Please don't touch my things." "I want to play a different game." "It's not funny to me. Please stop." "I'm not comfortable with that." "That's a secret I don't want to share." "I don't like being left out. Can we do something fair?" "I want to be treated kindly, please."

Boundaries show people how you want to be treated and help stop social conflict from escalating.

Developing our inner compass

Our feelings and body signals guide us towards safe, respectful friendships. This "inner compass" also warns us when a situation feels pressured, mean, or unsafe.

Hand out A4 paper or miniature whiteboards to each student. Project the Inner Compass poster on the board (Figure 9.2).

Inner compass reflection

Invite students to sit comfortably and follow the instructions with you.
Before choosing friends or handling tricky moments, we can listen to our
body and feelings—our inner compass always gives us clues.

Let's take a breath together.
Your Inner Compass helps you notice when a situation or friendship feels good (or not so good) for you. It helps you protect your boundaries and choose what's right and best for you.

Notice how your feelings change with different people—your inner compass helps you choose safe friendships and steer clear of those that need caution.

Ask your students
What do you think about the compass?
Do you see some feelings that would fit somewhere in between each of the four directions?

THE FRIENDSHIP BLUEPRINT

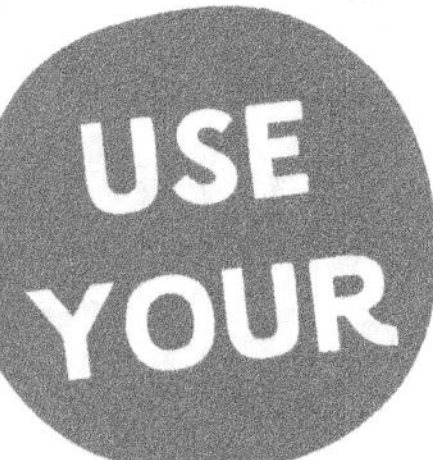

USE YOUR FRIENDSHIP COMPASS

N

THIS FRIENDSHIP FEELS GOOD FOR ME.

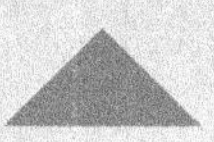

Your feelings and body help you know. Does this friendship feel kind, safe, and happy, or not?

W

I'M CONFUSED. I NEED SOME TIME TO THINK.

E

I NEED SOME SPACE NOW.

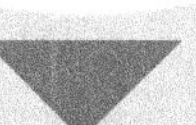

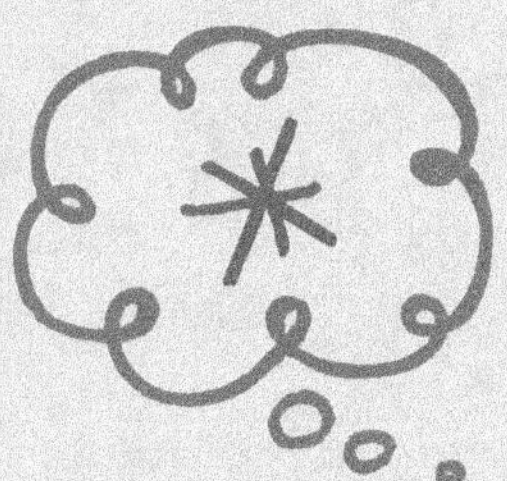

S

THIS FRIENDSHIP DOESN'T FEEL RIGHT FOR ME.

> **Where do you find yourself in the compass when you're:**
>
> Around someone who listens to you?
> Being pressured into doing something you don't want to do?
> Being pulled into conflict?
> Asking for space and not being given it?

Self-awareness reflection using my inner compass

Explain that self-awareness helps students choose their friends, set boundaries, and avoid unnecessary conflict. They can step back and choose what's right for them.

Display the inner compass in your classroom, and each day, help your students ask themselves:

"Where was my Inner Compass today? N, E, S, or W? What helped me feel
grounded?"
This builds ongoing self-awareness, boundaries, and social confidence.

Boundaries and the inner compass

Ask your students, *"What are your social boundaries?"* Some of them may still struggle to understand what social boundaries are, so you can help them by talking about how when someone does something that feels like an orange or red light, or like a south or west, that is probably a sign that their social boundaries have been crossed.

Everyone has social boundaries, and it's important to know yours. Examples of social boundaries include:

Not liking it when people ask for your opinion about a peer.
Feeling uncomfortable about being mean on purpose to someone.
Being asked to do something you don't want to do.
Breaking the school rules.
Not listening to parents or teachers.
Ignoring/excluding students.
Being asked to share personal information about yourself or others.

Ask students to reflect on their personal boundaries and encourage them to think carefully when those boundaries are crossed.

Boundaries role plays

The following role plays provide opportunities for students to reflect on their personal boundaries, how to set limits with friends when their expectations don't align with their values, and how to say "no." These role plays can be acted out or discussed in small groups or individually, including references to the inner compass where relevant. The role plays help children recognise the importance of red, orange, and green lights in friendships, develop social reasoning, and make values-based decisions about who they spend time with.

The rule breaker friend

You and your friend are playing at the park. Your friend suggests climbing over a high fence, even though there's a sign saying not to.

What would you do?
How do you feel when your friend encourages you to break rules?
What might happen if you go along with it?
What would a kind, sensible friend do instead?

The teasing friend

Your friend keeps teasing you about something you're proud of (like your artwork, new shoes, or a hobby). They say they're "just joking," but it hurts your feelings.

What could you say to your friend?
How do you know when a joke goes too far?
How does it feel to be treated like this?
What would a kind friend say or do in this situation?

The kind new friend

There's a new student in class who's friendly and kind, but not very popular. Your current friends advise against hanging out with them.

What do you do?
How do your current friends make you feel about your choices?

What does the new friend do that makes you feel safe and accepted?
Why is it important to mix with people who are kind, even if they're different?

The pushy friend

Your friend always wants things their way. If you disagree, they stop talking to you or say you're not being a good friend.

How does that make you feel?
Is it fair to only do what one person wants?
What can you say to stand up for yourself in a kind manner?
How would a respectful friend act differently?

The supportive friend

You make a mistake during a class presentation. One friend laughs and makes a joke, while another friend smiles and says, "You did your best!"

How do you feel about each friend's reaction?
Who helps you feel better about yourself?
Which friend would you want to be like?
Why is it important to choose supportive friends?

Practical ways to assert your boundaries

Setting boundaries is rarely easy and will usually evoke a range of uncomfortable emotions. Share the following framework with your students to discuss and invite them to add their own suggestions (Figure 9.3).

Finding friends that uplift well-being. (Self-Awareness, Empathy, and Perspective Taking)

Share the friendship choices poster with your class to help them ask themselves the right questions about friendships (Figure 9.4).

These reflection questions not only help students choose the **right friends** but also empower them to be the kind of **friend they want to have,** creating a foundation for lifelong, meaningful relationships.

SOMEONE CROSSED YOUR BOUNDARIES?
SPEAK UP & STAY STRONG

If someone makes you uncomfortable, be brave and speak up. Use these ways to protect your boundaries.

Say how you feel. "I feel upset when you take my things. Please ask next time."

Suggest something else. "I don't want to play that game. Want to play this one instead?"

Say "no" politely. "Thanks for asking, but I can't do that right now."

Say "no" without saying "no". "Not today," "Not now," "Maybe later," or "I need to think about it."

Share your feelings calmly. "I feel upset when you interrupt me. Can we take turns talking?"

Set a limit. "I can play for 10 more minutes, then I need a break."

Ask for space. "I need some quiet time. Let's talk later."

Find a compromise. "I don't want to do that, but maybe we can find something we both like?"

Say what's best for you. "I don't like being made fun of, even as a joke. Can we use kind words?"

Give a gentle reminder. "Remember, I don't like rough games. Can we play something else?"

Remind them. You like your friend, but not their behaviour. "I like hanging out with you, but I need to do this my way. Thanks for understanding."

FRIENDSHIP CHECK-IN
HOW TO BE A GREAT FRIEND

Do they take no for an answer?

Can I be myself with them?
Being yourself makes friendships awesome.

Do they treat people well?
Friends who are kind make everyone feel welcome.

Do they listen and care about my feelings?
Good friends listen, care, and cheer each other on.

Do I feel safe and accepted around them?
Safe friendships help me feel happy.

Do they make kind, respectful choices?
A real friend never makes me do something I don't want to.

How do I feel after spending time with them?
If I feel happy, that's a sign of a great friendship.

Do they say sorry or try to fix things when there's a problem?
Good friends fix mistakes and move on together.

Do they cheer me on when I do well?
Good friends celebrate together, not compete.

Do they gossip or try to get me to leave others out?
That's a red light, kind friends don't do that.

Do they help me be my best self?
Real friends help me grow and feel proud.

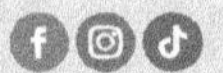

Joy check-in (Short Daily Practice)

Teaching children to *choose* relationships that support well-being does not happen in one or two lessons. Children need our support and guidance daily to remember the most helpful ways to work through their emotions.

At the end of each day, start the habit of sending your students home with a moment to reflect on what went well with their friendships.

"Who did you feel joyful with today?"
"What made that feel comfortable?"

This shifts the focus of friendship selection from popularity to feeling safe and sharing joy with one another.

The friendship tree

As adults, it's hard to watch students choose friends who aren't a good match for them. But belonging is a basic human need, and young people sometimes seek connection in the wrong places.

Friendships are complex, especially for young, developing minds. We can help by clearly teaching what to look for in a friend and encouraging kindness and respect.

Draw or print a large tree on the board with sturdy roots and branches. Students write foundational aspects of friendship in the trunk and roots, and add "good to have" qualities as leaves. In small groups, brainstorm as many strong friendship qualities as possible.

Bring the class together to complete the friendship tree, filling in qualities to look for in a friend.

The friendship compass

Provide students with an A4 piece of paper or open a fresh page in one of their books. Divide the page into 4 quadrants identified with the titles below:

Friendship qualities that lift me up.
Friendship qualities that pull me down.
Friendship qualities that help me be myself.
Friendship qualities I'm unsure about.

Next, students map the qualities of friendship they've experienced into the correct quadrant. Remind students not to name names, but to focus on the behaviours. Younger students can engage in this activity through a brainstorming session or by drawing pictures with simpler images you can design for them without words.

Friendship stars

Stars symbolise light. Remind students they can bring positivity and kindness to others, helping create happier, more connected schools (Fredrickson, 2001).

Draw a big star on the board and give each student a star cutout. Brainstorm words and actions that bring light to friendships. Ask students to write how they bring warmth and joy to their friendships on their star, and display them in the classroom or their well-being books.

Younger students enjoy being called "friendship stars," while older students may prefer "be the light."

Reflect often on this concept to help students remember that we all carry a light within us and have a choice to share it or keep it to ourselves. Compliment students when you see them being the light, especially if it's to uplift others who are sitting in the darker moments of life.

Friendship star list and letters

After the friendship star activity, share a story about a friend who brought light to your life. Highlight their qualities with a specific example.

Encourage students to value friendships beyond school. Have them list five friends outside of school who bring them light, then write letters of appreciation highlighting the qualities they're grateful for. Help students deliver these letters with their caregivers' support.

Would you choose this friend? (Self-Awareness, Communication Skills, Empathy and Perspective Taking)

It can be hard to see clearly when you're in the middle of a friendship. Use role-plays or shows like Little Lunch and Bluey to examine situations objectively. After watching, discuss which friend students would choose and why, then move into role-play activities.

Role plays

Have students pair up.

Read or act out each situation. For every scenario, ask: What would a kind friend say? An unkind friend? Have pairs act out both responses to build awareness of supportive and unsupportive friendship behaviours.

Social situations to role play

You trip in front of your class.

You're picked last for a team.

You come last in a relay race.

You fall off the monkey bars and scream so loud, it feels like half your school is standing around you. You're crying a lot, but there isn't a scratch or bruise that anyone can see, and you're embarrassed.

You tripped over a friend's jigsaw puzzle that they just finished. It's broken badly.

You're on stage with your class for the school musical. The nerves take over, and you can hardly breathe. You're scared, and you run off the stage.

Your teacher asks you to solve a Maths problem in front of the class, but Maths is your hardest subject. You don't know how to answer it, and you're really embarrassed.

You are the only one in your class who doesn't know their timetables.

It's Special Visitors' Day at your school, and no one from your family is coming.

You're waiting in line for the canteen, and just as you get to the counter, you realise you left your money at home.

You miss the winning goal for your team in soccer.

Your parents have changed their minds about getting a puppy for your family.

Afterwards, discuss as a group the impact of kind and unkind responses.

Relational aggression (social conflict that involves deliberate manipulation and friendship sabotage). (Conflict Resolution and Problem Solving, Empathy and Perspective Taking, Communication Skills)

Social conflict is a normal part of growing up, especially as emotions fluctuate (Crick & Dodge, 1994; Rose & Rudolph, 2006).

The Friendship Blueprint addresses rising conflict and relational aggression in primary school—a stage when children begin to value peers' opinions more than adults' (Benish-Weisman et al., 2021).

Relational aggression, once common in teenagers, is now seen in children as young as eight (Grotpeter & Crick, 1996).

Today's children also carry the burden of pandemic-related anxiety and rapid social change (Loades et al., 2020). Social media and mobile phones, designed to be addictive, increase social challenges (Livingstone & Smith, 2014; Ortutay, 2023b). Despite parents' best efforts, it's difficult to set healthy technology boundaries (Odgers & Jensen, 2020).

Children now use phones to arrange social events and resolve conflicts by text, which can make problems worse. Well-meaning parental involvement can unintentionally amplify children's social upsets, making it harder for them to develop confidence in managing their own friendships.

How can adults help children avoid friendship roadblocks? At this age, emotions often override logic, making it hard to process social upsets calmly. Children need support to manage these challenges.

Emotional intelligence and healthy boundaries develop over time. Social conflicts often stem from misunderstandings and strong emotions. The Friendship Blueprint gives students tools to regulate emotions, increase self-awareness, and respond pro-socially, even if mistakes still happen.

Navigating social conflict and relational aggression isn't easy, but it's possible. The tools in this lesson equip young people to respond proactively and pro-socially.

Getting your facts right

Often, social conflict arises from misunderstandings and miscommunication. Social conflict can quickly lead to overthinking and anxiety. We're wired to feel concerned when something is up within our social group because we're a social species that relies on each other to thrive. Anxious thoughts that cascade out of our survival brains are rarely true, yet they often feel completely true. All too often, other children get involved, and suddenly there is a big social commotion with very little basis in fact.

Discuss this with your students and explain how emotions can take over during social conflicts. When emotions are high, our thinking capacity is low. Ask your students if they can think of a time they got their facts wrong and wasted a lot of time worrying about a situation they didn't need to?

There are often multiple explanations for why someone behaves a certain way, and jumping to conclusions and filling in the gaps without enough facts will almost always magnify the issue.

Getting my facts straight: Role plays

Challenge students to create their own role-plays about social conflicts that escalate due to misunderstandings or assumptions. Encourage creativity and humour.

Here are some ways to get your facts straight to help resolve a friendship drama where a lot of the facts are unavailable or imagined:

"I noticed you were quiet today. Are you okay?"

"Can I check something with you? I just want to make sure I've got this right."

"When you said/did XYZ, what did you mean by that?"

"I might have misunderstood. Can you tell me what happened from your point of view?"

"I've been feeling a bit unsure about what's going on between us. Can we talk it through?"

"Did I do something that upset you, or is there something else going on?"

"I don't want to assume anything. Can you help me understand what really happened?"

"Is everything okay between us, or have I got the wrong idea?"

"Can we clear something up? I heard/noticed something and want to make sure it's true before I worry about it."

"Would you mind explaining how you felt about what happened? I want to understand better."

"I care about our friendship, and I'd rather ask you directly than guess. Can we talk about it?"

"Did you mean to leave me out, or was it a mistake?"

"What you said really upset me. Did you mean that the way it sounded?"

"Could you please say that again? I want to make sure I understood properly."

"Are you okay? I had a funny feeling you weren't feeling good about something."

"It looked like you were looking right at me when you whispered and laughed with our group earlier. Is that what happened, or am I worrying about nothing?"

Once the role plays have come to an end, find a place to display these questions to continue helping guide students through miscommunications and misunderstandings that can amplify conflict.

The following conversation tips will help your students find the words to get facts right.

Getting the facts straight: A friendship conversation guide

When we don't have all the facts, small problems can grow. Asking kind, curious questions is better than jumping to conclusions or making assumptions.

Here are some tips to extend your conversation to fact-check with your friend.

1. **Your tone matters.** If you say any of the kind and curious statements with an angry voice, you won't get your message across in a way that makes your friend feel safe and comfortable enough to listen. Keep your voice calm and friendly.
2. **Use "I" statements** instead of "you" (e.g., "I felt unsure" instead of "You made me feel…").
3. **Smile** or use gentle eye contact if that feels comfortable.
4. **Calm yourself.** Take a few slow breaths. Remind yourself: "I'm trying to understand, not accuse."
5. **Choose a good time** and a calm tone to talk to your friend.
6. **Start the conversation kindly.** Use one of the sentence starters from earlier, like, "Hey, can I ask you something? I just want to make sure I understand."
7. **Ask clarifying questions** (Be curious, don't blame). "When you said/did ___, what did you mean?" "Can you tell me what actually happened from your point of view?" "Is everything okay between us, or did I do something that bothered you?" "I heard something and wanted to check if it's true before I get worried." "How were you feeling when that happened?"
8. **Listen and reflect.** Really listen and don't interrupt. Try to see things from their side. Say things like: "Thanks for telling me that." "I didn't realise, that makes sense now." "I appreciate you being honest."
9. **Find a way forward.** You can finish with something positive: "I'm glad we talked about it." "Let's move on and keep being honest with each other." "Next time, I'll check in sooner instead of worrying."

Thank students for their creativity in role-plays and praise their efforts to build positive relationships and reduce relational aggression.

Online communication for connection and to avoid social conflict and relational aggression

Many young people communicate with friends online in various ways, including through gaming, text messages, and social media. Back in the day, when mobile phones were not used by children, going home provided a safe harbour from social roadblocks and relational aggression, allowing time to think, cool off, and come up with a plan for the next day. Young people who use devices to communicate miss out on the much-needed break from peers to enjoy their own company, spend time with family, pursue hobbies, and get some fresh air without the drama.

Conflict can grow rapidly via texting, where tone and facial expressions are removed from the equation, leaving children to rely solely on the written word and the intensity of their emotions. Further to this, whatever they write can't be unwritten and can be read by anyone else, including other children and parents.

Remind your students that our words matter and that our communication should be positive to create a safe and fruitful social world. Project the "Online? Be kind. Have fun and stay safe," and remind them again that what they post online stays online. It would also be a good idea to share these guidelines in your newsletter, or even add them to your policies, crediting it as "The Friendship Blueprint by Madhavi Nawana Parker © 2026 Routledge, London." This way, you are spreading the boundaries as far and wide as possible to help children follow them easily.

Enhance the discussion further, with the following points, encouraging deeper student led exploration.

Important rules to remember when texting online

Think before you send

Once you hit send, you can't take it back. Ask yourself: "Would I say this to their face?" and "Would I want my family to receive a message like this?"

Use words that feel friendly, not fiery

Tone can get lost in texts. A joke can sound mean without your smile or voice. Add kindness with emojis or gentle words like "no worries" or "thanks for explaining."

If it's private, keep it private

Don't share someone's messages, photos, or secrets without asking first. Trust is difficult to rebuild once it has been broken.

Pause before you reply when you're upset

If you're feeling angry or hurt, take a moment to step back. Wait, breathe, and come back to it later when you're calm.

Be clear and kind

Short texts can be misunderstood. Use full sentences or kind clarifiers: "I didn't mean that in a bad way."

Include others, don't exclude them online

Avoid starting group chats or posts that intentionally exclude someone. Inclusion online matters just as much as it does in person.

Protect your personal information

Never share your full name, address, school, passwords, or private photos. Keep your digital footprint safe.

Don't forward or screenshot hurtful things

If someone sends you something unkind or private, don't pass it on. It can hurt people and cause real harm.

Be your real self online

Stay true to who you are. It's easy to hide behind a screen, but real friends like you for your honesty (Figure 9.5).

Role plays: Digital conflict

Divide your group into pairs or trios to role-play a digital conflict. Younger students may not need this; however, you may offer it at your discretion.

ONLINE?

BE KIND, HAVE FUN, AND STAY SAFE.

Text to make plans or share smiles, **not to argue.**

Got a problem? Call or chat in person!

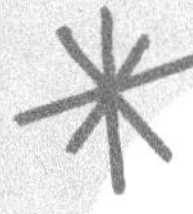

Stop and think before you post. Is it kind? Is it true? Is it needed? Only share if yes.

Give real compliments, share friendly jokes, and **make others smile**.

If you're upset, pause, put your device down, count to ten, or ask an adult for help.

Always ask before sharing photos or messages, **respect others' privacy**.

Group chats. **Include everyone** and keep it kind. If it turns mean, leave or speak up kindly.

Use kind emojis to share happy feelings. **Don't use emojis to tease** or be mean.

Take breaks from screens, move, play, and **talk with friends in person**.

Only share what's true, kind, and safe. Don't spread rumours or secrets.

Be kind online and offline, everyone has feelings, just like you.

If something feels wrong, tell a trusted adult. **You're never alone.**

I have met many preschoolers who use text-to-speech and audio-to-text to leave messages for playmates.

Students will create their own role plays using the following problem-solving goals to improve outcomes after a digital mishap.

Problem-solving goals: Digital kindness. Apologising online and offline. Understanding the impact of online actions. Expressing feelings calmly. Asking questions rather than making assumptions. Listening to each other's perspectives. Repairing trust.

After each Role Play, ask the class the following questions:

What could have been done differently?
How can we promote greater inclusivity online?
How could the hurt friend speak up kindly?
What can the others do to show they care?
How can they include each other next time?

Remind your students about the value of assertive communication, which involves:

Staying curious and non-judgmental.
Giving others a chance to explain.
Apologising and making it right.
Finding a respectful way to raise an issue.
Repairing trust.
Being brave enough to be accountable and make things better.

Now your students have explored the social dangers of text and online communication, remind them how important it is to keep going back over those online and text rules, perhaps even keeping them nearby at home to make sure they stay kind, respectful, and safe, leaving a positive digital footprint they can be proud of.

To further support students in primary and high school to understand the importance of online safety, I highly recommend starting with: https://www.esafety.gov.au/ and also, for powerful presentations on e-safety I recommend Wayne Holdsworth from Smack talk: https://smacktalk.com.au/ and Susan McLean https://www.inspirespeakers.com.au/speakers/show/susan-mclean/

Wise ways to avoid relational aggression. (Conflict Resolution and Problem Solving, Self-Awareness, Communication Skills)

Young people have much to learn in today's fast-paced social world. The more they know, the better they can manage the emotional pain of conflict.

What is relational aggression?

Relational aggression is when someone uses friendships, social power, manipulation, and friendship sabotage to hurt others. It's not about hitting or yelling, and it's much more subtle. It's about using relationships to exclude, control, or harm feelings. Relational aggression can be more common in triads where three people are in a social group, with one person holding power and assuming the highest social position (Browne & Carroll-Lind, 2006). The other two group members are often found trying to please the most powerful friend, who will play them off against each other to keep them both in the highest, most powerful positions. Relational aggression can, of course, happen in any-sized group or between two children. Here are some examples seen in primary schools around the world:

Leaving someone out on purpose.
Spreading rumours or gossip.
Giving the silent treatment.
Saying "You can't be my friend unless…"
Turning other people against someone.

These behaviours hurt deeply and can cause long-lasting harm to someone's self-esteem and emotional safety (Demirel, 2020; Espelage & Swearer, 2010; Olweus, 1993; Rubin et al., 2015).

Help your students understand what relational aggression is and express how you will call it out when you see it, and that you want to know when it's happening in your community. Children need to know we are upholding a high standard of social conduct for everyone's benefit. Simple definitions include:

"Relational aggression is when someone uses friendship to hurt others."
"Relational aggression is using popularity, gossip, exclusion, or silence to control people or cause social harm."

Help your students understand the warning signs that someone is going through it, and discuss afterwards how they would feel if they were experiencing this.

Warning signs

They suddenly don't want to go to school or hang out.
They don't seem themselves.
They are alone during play breaks, even though they are usually with people.
They seem anxious about group chats or social events.
They say things like, "No one likes me," or "Everyone's mad at me, but I don't know why."

Invite your students to share how they would feel if they were experiencing relational aggression. Then open a discussion to explore the following points for discussion to help eliminate relational aggression.

Say no to relational aggression. It's not cool to be cruel

Relational aggression is when someone uses friendship to hurt others, using popularity, gossip, exclusion, or silence to control people or cause social harm. Here are some ways to stop relational aggression at our school:

Include, don't exclude.
  Invite others into games or conversations. Avoid saying, "You can't sit with us." If the person is doing something hurtful, and that's why you don't want them to join them, explain it in a kind way or ask an adult for help. Kindness is contagious.
Stop gossip in its tracks
  If someone shares something personal, keep it private and don't talk about people who aren't with you at the time.
Use words to solve problems and talk directly to the person you are having an upset with.

  "I felt left out when you made plans without me. Can we talk about it?"

Speak up or walk away.
  If you see others being hurt, say something:

  "That's not cool," or "She's my friend too."

Or simply walk away, don't get involved and report it to an adult.

Think before you post or comment

Ask: "Is this kind? "Would I say this face-to-face? "How would I feel if this were said about me?"

Be Open to Feedback

If someone tells you that your actions hurt them, take a moment to reflect. You can say:

"I didn't realise that hurt you. I'll try to do better."

Owning your behaviour takes strength.

Be kind. Everyone has a story. We never know what someone is going through, and we should always be kind.

> **REMEMBER.**
> *Relational aggression is real, and it hurts.*
> *You can choose kindness, even when others don't.*
> *Friendship is built on safety, kindness, and respect.*
> *If someone treats others badly, they may treat you that way too. Choose friends who treat people well.*

Relational aggression posters

Allow students time to work in groups to create posters that reflect the previous discussion in their own words, adding their own insights. Display these posters as content refreshers.

Relational aggression role plays

Help your students form pairs or small groups, using the poster guidelines to respond in a friendly, constructive way.

The whispering circle

A group of friends is whispering and looking at someone while laughing. The left-out person notices and feels hurt.

Roles: The group of friends, the person left out, a bystander.
Goal: Practice speaking up, including others, and repairing trust.
Reflection: *How would you feel in this situation? What could the bystander do?*

"You can't be friends with her"

A friend tells you not to hang out with another person, or you'll be left out, too.

Roles: The controlling friend, the person caught in the middle, the other friend.
Goal: Practice setting boundaries and staying true to your values.
Reflection: *How can you handle peer pressure without being unkind?*

Group chat exclusion

A group chat is made for everyone, except one person, who finds out.

Roles: The person excluded, someone in the group chat, a friend who noticed.
Goal: Practice empathy and repair online behaviours.
Reflection: *What are the real-life impacts of digital exclusion?*

Secret sharing

You told a friend something personal. Now others know, and you're embarrassed.

Roles: The person who shared the secret, the friend who told others, and another friend who witnessed it.
Goal: Practice repairing trust and understanding consequences.
Reflection: *How can friendships recover from broken trust?*

"You can't sit with us"

A new student asks to join a group at lunch and is told there's no room.

Roles: The excluded student, the group members, a teacher, or a bystander.
Goal: Practice inclusion and kindness in public spaces.
Reflection: *How does exclusion affect someone's sense of belonging?*

Eye rolls and silent treatment

One friend starts ignoring another and rolling their eyes whenever they speak.

Roles: The friend being ignored, the one doing it, a mutual friend.
Goal: Explore non-verbal relational aggression and repair strategies.
Reflection: *How can silent behaviours cause harm?*

The group turned against one person

One person in a friend group starts spreading negative stories to turn the group against someone.

Roles: The person targeted, the person spreading things, and others in the group.
Goal: Practice speaking up and choosing not to join hurtful behaviour.
Reflection: *What does real loyalty look like in friendship?*

Partners picked last on purpose

A class is doing partner work, and a student is always left last because others say they're "too weird" or "too slow."

Roles: The excluded student, classmates, and teacher.
Goal: Practice inclusive thinking and changing group culture.
Reflection: *What message are we sending when we exclude someone?*

Making fun of interests

Scenario: A friend is mocked for liking something different (e.g., anime, bugs, books).
Roles: The friend being teased, the teaser, a bystander who supports or stays silent.
Goal: Explore acceptance and personal boundaries.
Reflection: *How do we create space for people to be themselves?*

Fake compliments

A friend says, "You look great today—for once," and laughs. Everyone laughs along.

Roles: The person insulted, the one giving the comment, and the friends laughing.
Goal: Discuss sarcasm, backhanded compliments, and emotional safety.
Reflection: *Is it still funny if someone's feelings are hurt?*

These role plays work best when followed by open-ended discussion, opportunities for reflection, or journaling.

Choosing to be the kind of friend I want to have

Discuss how "The Friendship Blueprint" has helped students make better friendship choices. Brainstorm what to look for in a friend. Then, have students reflect and write or draw about the kind of friend they were, are, and want to be. Remind them that kindness, understanding, and good boundaries help everyone.

As you close this chapter, thank your students for their hard work in creating a Friendship Blueprint for your school.

Share improvements you've noticed in well-being and class culture. Ask students if the school feels different and what more can be done.

Close with a celebration or small surprise to show your pride in students' progress. Create certificates to recognise their work on friendships and their growth into kind, authentic friends.

Finally, to you, the educator: thank you for choosing this work to enhance your own. Your dedication and effort in a changing educational landscape are deeply respected.

You are leaders and changemakers. Your impact is far-reaching and invaluable. Here's to you, your students, and positive school communities everywhere.

With warmest wishes always, Madhavi

Key takeaways from Chapter 9

- The friends you choose shape your wellbeing, confidence, and sense of belonging.
- Setting boundaries and listening to your inner compass helps you choose friends who support your growth.
- Real friends let you be yourself, include others, repair mistakes, and communicate kindly, both online and in person.
- Relational aggression and social conflict can be effectively addressed through empathy, problem-solving, and respectful communication.
- Everyone deserves safe, uplifting friendships, and you can contribute to a positive school culture by being a "friendship star."

Call to action

Be a Friendship Hero! Every day, make a choice to be kind, include others, and look for ways to brighten someone's day. If you see someone left out, invite them in. If you notice a friend feeling down, cheer them up. Together, you can make your school the happiest and safest place to be.

Help students be intentional about the friendships they build and the kind of friend they choose to be. Teach students to pause, get perspective, and choose peace over drama. Develop a shared language and response plan for managing the ups and downs of friendships, so students feel equipped to navigate social challenges without harm. Each day, look for ways to include, uplift, and show empathy to your colleagues so you're modelling what you expect from your students. You have the power to make your classroom and community a safer, happier place for everyone.

References

Allen, K., & Bowles, T. (2012). Belonging as a guiding principle in the education of adolescents. *Australian Journal of Educational & Developmental Psychology, 12,* 108–119.

Antonopoulou, K., Chaidemenou, A., & Kouvava, S. (2019). Peer acceptance and friendships among primary school pupils: Associations with loneliness, self-esteem and school engagement. *Educational Psychology in Practice, 35*(3), 339–351. https://eric.ed.gov/?id=EJ1223292

Bagwell, C. L., & Schmidt, M. E. (2011). *Friendships in childhood and adolescence.* The Guilford Press.

Bauminger-Zviely, N. (2013). Social and academic abilities in children with high functioning autism spectrum disorder: Peer relations, loneliness and classroom climate. *Journal of Autism and Developmental Disorders, 43,* 1157–1172.

Benish-Weisman, M., Oreg, S., & Berson, Y. (2021). The contribution of peer values to children's values and behavior. *Personality and Social Psychology Bulletin, 48*(6), 014616722110201. https://doi.org/10.1177/01461672211020193

Blakemore, S.-J., & Mills, K. L. (2014). Is adolescence a sensitive period for sociocultural processing? *Annual Review of Psychology, 65,* 187–207.

Browne, J., & Carroll-Lind, J. (2006). Relational aggression between primary school girls. *Kairaranga, 7*(1), 20–29. https://doi.org/10.54322/kairaranga.v7i1.41

Bukowski, W. M., Laursen, B., & Rubin, K. H. (2018). *Handbook of peer interactions, relationships, and groups* (2nd ed.). Guilford Press.

CASEL. (2020). *What is the CASEL framework?* CASEL; Collaborative for Academic, Social, and Emotional Learning (CASEL). https://casel.org/fundamentals-of-sel/what-is-the-casel-framework/

Crick, N. R., & Dodge, K. A. (1994). A review and reformulation of social information-processing mechanisms in children's social adjustment. *Psychological Bulletin, 115*(1), 74–101.

Demirel, Ö. Ü. Y. (2020). Model proposal for preventing relational aggression in schools. *International Social Sciences Studies Journal, 6*(71), 4503–4513. http://dx.doi.org/10.26449/sssj.2704

Durlak, J. A., Weissberg, R. P., Dymnicki, A. B., Taylor, R. D., & Schellinger, K. B. (2011). The impact of enhancing students' social and emotional learning: a meta-analysis of school-based universal interventions. *Child Development, 82*(1), 405–432.https://doi.org/10.1111/j.1467-8624.2010.01564.x

Espelage, D. L., & Swearer, S. M. (2010). A social-ecological model for bullying prevention and intervention: Understanding the impact of peers, schools, families, and communities. In S. R. Jimerson, S. M. Swearer, & D. L. Espelage (Eds.), *Handbook of bullying in schools: An international perspective* (pp. 61–72). Routledge.

Fredrickson, B. L. (2001). The role of positive emotions in positive psychology: The broaden-and-build theory of positive emotions. *American Psychologist, 56*(3), 218–226.

Grotpeter, J. K., & Crick, N. R. (1996). Relational aggression, overt aggression, and friendship. *Child Development, 67*(5), 2328–2338. https://pubmed.ncbi.nlm.nih.gov/9022244/

Güroğlu, B. (2022b). The power of friendship: The developmental significance of friendships from a neuroscience perspective. *Child Development Perspectives, 16*(2), 110–117. https://doi.org/10.1111/cdep.12450

Livingstone, S., & Smith, P. K. (2014). Annual research review: Harms experienced by child users of online and mobile technologies: The nature, prevalence and management of sexual and aggressive risks in the digital age. *Journal of Child Psychology and Psychiatry, 55*(6), 635–654. https://doi.org/10.1111/jcpp.12197

Loades, M. E., Chatburn, E., Higson-Sweeney, N., Reynolds, S., Shafran, R., Brigden, A., Linney, C., McManus, M. N., Borwick, C., & Crawley, E. (2020). Rapid systematic review: the impact of social isolation and loneliness on the mental health of children and adolescents in the context of COVID-19. *Journal of the American Academy of Child & Adolescent Psychiatry, 59*(11), 1218–1239. https://doi.org/10.1016/j.jaac.2020.05.009

Odgers, C. L., & Jensen, M. R. (2020). Annual research review: Adolescent mental health in the digital age: facts, fears, and Future Directions. *Journal of Child Psychology and Psychiatry, 61*(3), 336–348. https://doi.org/10.1111/jcpp.13190

Olweus, D. (1993). *Bullying at school: What we know and what we can do*. Wiley-Blackwell.

Ortutay, B. (2023b, October 24). *States sue Meta claiming its social platforms are addictive and harm children's mental health*. AP News. https://apnews.com/article/metachildrenteensharmslawsuit-17858802d76143d358e38ee15150dc94

Rose, A. J., & Rudolph, K. D. (2006). A review of sex differences in peer relationship processes: Potential trade-offs for the emotional and behavioral development of girls and boys. *Psychological Bulletin, 132*(1), 98–131. https://doi.org/10.1037/0033-2909.132.1.98

Rubin, K. H., Bukowski, W. M., & Bowker, J. C. (2015). Children in peer groups. In M. H. Bornstein, T. Leventhal, & R. M. Lerner (Eds.), *Handbook of child psychology and developmental science: Ecological settings and processes* (7th ed., pp. 175–222). John Wiley & Sons, Inc.

Steinberg, L., & Monahan, K. C. (2007). Age differences in resistance to peer influence. *Developmental Psychology, 43*(6), 1531–1543. https://doi.org/10.1037/0012-1649.43.6.1531

Swedell, L. (2012). *Primate sociality and social systems*. Nature.com. https://www.nature.com/scitable/knowledge/library/primate-sociality-and-social-systems-58068905/

Waite, C. (2021). *Peer connections reimagined: Innovations nurturing student networks to unlock opportunity*. https://files.eric.ed.gov/fulltext/ED614146.pdf

Wentzel, K. R., & Caldwell, K. (1997). Friendships, peer acceptance, and group membership: relations to academic achievement in middle school. *Child Development, 68*(6), 1198–1209. https://doi.org/10.1111/j.1467-8624.1997.tb01994.x

Appendix: Friendship activities and games

To make learning about friendship even more fun, try these activities at school or at home:

1. **Friendship quest challenge:** Create a checklist of daily or weekly friendship missions (e.g., "Invite someone new to play," "Give a genuine compliment"). Earn points for each completed mission!
2. **Friendship comic strip:** Draw a comic about a friendship adventure or a tricky social situation and how you solved it.
3. **Kindness chain:** Start a paper chain in your classroom. Each link represents a kind act—see how long you can make it together!
4. **Compliment jar:** Write kind messages to classmates and add them to the jar. Read some aloud each week.
5. **Friendship bingo:** Make a bingo card with positive friendship actions. Mark off each one you do.

Keep exploring, creating, and sharing! The more you practice friendship skills, the stronger and happier your classroom will become.

Final note

Here we are, at the end of The Friendship Blueprint.

Thank you for reading.

Thank you for believing.

Thank you for joining me for the ride.

I hope this book has been everything you hoped for and more. Further training is available at www.positivemindsaustralia.com.au and you can follow along on social media here

Figure FN.1 QR code link to social media

I wish you and your students the very best of everything, especially friendships, always.

Madhavi

Index